Nursing the Psychiatric Emergency

Nursing the Psychiatric Emergency

Martin F. Ward
RMN DN RNT Cert. Ed. NEBSS Dip. M. Phil.

Research Fellow – Mental Health,
National Institute for Nursing, Oxford;
Nursing Research Advisor,
Oxford Mental Health Care NHS Trust

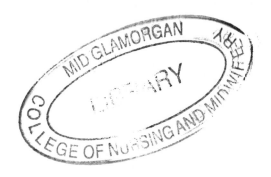
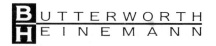
BUTTERWORTH HEINEMANN

Butterworth-Heinemann Ltd
Linacre House, Jordan Hill, Oxford OX2 8DP

℞   A member of the Reed Elsevier group

OXFORD   LONDON   BOSTON
MUNICH   NEW DELHI   SINGAPORE   SYDNEY
TOKYO   TORONTO   WELLINGTON

First published 1995

British Library Cataloguing in Publication Data

A catalogue record for this book is available from the British Library.

ISBN 0 7506 1592 3

Composition by Scribe Design, Gillingham, Kent, UK
Printed in Great Britain by Biddles Ltd, Guildford and Kings Lynn

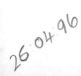

26.04.96

Contents

Preface

The first day I started clinical work as a student psychiatric nurse a man cut his wrists in the toilet. He had not been missed for nearly half an hour, and consequently had lost a considerable amount of blood. I was asked to clear it up. I remember standing there looking at the aftermath of this man's pain and frustration, desperately wanting to help in some way but feeling totally useless. What was worse was that I had no idea how to clear up the blood, and because everyone else appeared to be doing things which seemed far more important I did not feel I could ask for help. I made a complete mess of the job and was subsequently ridiculed for my apparent ineptitude by the hardened nursing veterans who made up the rest of the team. Protesting that no-one had told me how to clear up such things was simply met with derision. I went home that night feeling pretty miserable. I spoke to a friend about it who insisted that if I wanted to end my career before it had even begun, on the basis of one very minor episode, perhaps I should not have started in the first place. That was all the support I got. The trouble was that even though what he said made sense, and even though my part in the episode was almost inconsequential, I still felt a failure.

That was 1969, but I have never forgotten that day. What it taught me was that no matter how well prepared you think you are there is always the possibility that you will be called upon to do something for which you were unprepared. If you are a nurse, or a member of the caring professions, the possibility of such events occurring increases considerably. Those people who are the most vulnerable, i.e. the unqualified, the unsupported and the unskilled, are the ones who are most at risk. Yet everyone who works with clients who have problems with mental health must face the possibility of being challenged by events and behaviours which may frighten, confuse or threaten them.

This book deals with the Psychiatric Emergency (PE) from a healthcare professional's point of view. It looks at the events and situations which may constitute such episodes and formulates approaches that may be used in extreme times. A systematic framework for approaching such events (AIRS) is discussed and its components of assessment, intervention, resolution and support are applied to a series of different clinical examples.

The first part of the book compares issues of crisis with those of emergency and explains the two concepts. Professional coping strategies and emergency psychiatric nursing are considered next, and examples of PEs are given in a variety of clinical settings, both residential and community. The central part of the book explores different types of PEs and looks at intervention principles appropriate to such events. Finally, issues of support, both individual and organizational, are discussed with recommendations for good practice. The whole is intended to provide information to individual care professionals about the nature, style and presentation of effective interventions that can be used in any psychiatric emergency situation. As such, the book is not intended for any one particular discipline, though those who deal more regularly with clients who suffer mental health problems will find the work most pertinent.

The reader should not regard the interventions used within the book as the only way of tackling the PE. They are described within the context of the AIRS framework as one alternative, to guide and inform. It is important that care workers devise their own intervention strategies, based upon their strengths and the principles contained herein. The framework has been developed as a way of bringing together the most contemporary information on PE management. However, I should like to thank the staff of both the Oxford and Norfolk Mental Health Care NHS Trusts whose experiences have informed the development of the text generally. Having the confidence and experience to know what to do when faced by extraordinary circumstances is a quality admired by most. Nurses and healthcare professionals are expected to have this quality in abundance, yet the reality is they are often asked to do things beyond their skills base or their experience. Unfortunately, they do not have the luxury of being able to call upon someone else to help them out in such situations because invariably it is the very nature of their work which makes them the last 'line of defence'. It is because I can remember so vividly what happened to me on my first day in nursing, and because I know that so many people experience similar and often far more serious PEs, that this book is dedicated to every nurse who finds themself in a situation for which they were never prepared.

M.F.W.
Oxford, 1995

Author's note

Throughout the book I have tried to refer to the gender of clients and nurses as realistically as possible, i.e. him/herself, s/he etc. However, with the exception of some of the examples used in the book, where this would have made the text messy, or complicated, I have referred to the nurse as female and the client as male. This is, I know, unsatisfactory, but as yet no one has discovered a more acceptable alternative.

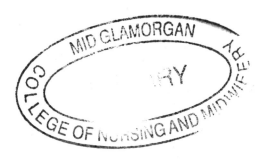

1

Emergency theory

Introduction

Have you ever found yourself in a situation which you had absolutely no idea how to handle? Have you ever been asked a probing and personal question for which you had no answer? Have you ever wished that the ground would swallow you up to save you from your embarrassment? Most of us, of course, have suffered such indignities, but somehow we manage to cope. However, our method of success is seldom considered after the event for we are usually too grateful to have come through to reflect upon what took place.

This ability that most of us have that allows us to deal with even the most difficult situations is an important part of our will to survive, and it is essential if we are to lead satisfactory and rewarding lives. We tend to see this apparent innate skill as being attractive, recognizing it in others and congratulating ourselves on our spontaneity and responsiveness. The only problem with such an approach is that if we do not learn from our experiences, or fail to plan for our failures, then there will be very little we can do when confronted by a real emergency.

For nurses, and not just those working in psychiatry, this poses a serious dilemma. On the one hand they must be natural, approachable and spontaneous, while on the other they must be professional, clear-headed and objective. For most of their working lives they would expect to use a combination of subjective and objective approaches to maintain the quality of their client–nurse relationships. Contemporary practice encourages clients and nurses to collaborate in care activities and, perhaps as a consequence of this, offers less potential for many of the difficult interpersonal problems traditionally associated with psychiatry. However, the very nature of their work suggests that at some time during their career nurses must expect to have to deal with a difficult, dangerous or even life-threatening situation.

Is it possible, at such times, to continue being spontaneous, natural and subjective? Probably not, though many competent nurses are capable of appearing 'cool, calm and collected' no matter what the situation. Is it acceptable to do 'what comes naturally' on such occasions? If this means muddling through in the vain hope that the problem will be resolved as if by magic, with no plan, no idea of personal effectiveness, and no hope of success, then the answer is a definite no.

The pressure to be successful is great, with nurses being well aware that their colleagues expect them to be able to cope effectively. However, it is not just the nursing profession which has high expectations of itself; society in general perceives nurses as being somehow different from the ordinary man or woman in the street. The attributes associated with the 'angel' include such things as compassion, sensitivity and understanding, but above all else the ability to cope effectively with anything and everything that happens to both them and their clients. Here lies the route cause of the dilemma, for the fact is that nurses are no different from anyone else. What distinguishes them is their professional education and the exposure to pain and suffering which clinical practice brings. Their coping abilities are often mythical, yet all too often nurses believe their own publicity and suffer severely when this is proven to be false.

The reality is that psychiatric nursing remains a difficult and complicated job. Psychiatric clients, no matter where they may be found, are often unpredictable, frightened and distressed; they may be prone to hurting themselves or others and frequently require assistance in meeting even the simplest of their personal needs. The irony is that twentieth-century enlightenment may have produced better working relationships between clients and nurses during the normal course of events, but when fear or an increase in psychological disturbance motivates the client to do something out of the ordinary, nurses may well find themselves in a situation which requires them to provide an extraordinary response. What happens to care-sharing at this point? What use is primary nursing when a client is threatening to kill themselves? How does a care philosophy stop a severely distressed man from strangling his wife in the middle of the out-patient clinic? More significantly, where do the skills come from for the nurse to be able to deal with these situations?

The answer should lie in the content of their professional education, and often the nucleus for it does. Unfortunately, all too often many nurses, and not just those working with the mentally ill, find themselves in client–nurse encounters for which they have never been prepared. The nature and style of their educational programme may influence the decisions they make but it cannot hope to see them through the reality of a life-threatening situation for which they may have total responsibility for the very first time. How can it support them through the self-doubt or rejection that accompanies failure, or the embarrassment that indecision causes them when others are watching. The simple answer is that professional preparation cannot accomplish any of these, and it is important that nurses recognize this if they are going to do anything about it.

Developing an approach

Some nurses, just like anyone else, appear to be able to deal with everything that happens to them; some have difficulty with certain difficult situations but not others, while a few do not seem to be able to handle anything unless they are given specific guidelines and are continuously supervised. What is it that causes these differences in ability, when the educational background and preparation for most nurses would be reasonably similar? Talley and Chiverton (1983) point to the importance of clinicians working in high stress areas being able to make connections between medical and psychiatric issues, while Cahill *et al.* (1991) state that psychiatric nurses must be able to function well under stress if they are going to initiate effective care. Similarly, Blomhoff *et al.* (1990) feel that some nurses are able to predict changes in the needs of their clients better than others because of the significance nurses place on accurate observation and assessment. These, and other authors, seem to suggest that the key to successful intervention during an emergency is preparation and planning, but few authors, if any, identify the nature and timing of either.

Another primary factor is the ability of the nurse to deal effectively with stress. Stress is often generated because the individual feels that they cannot cope, or can see no logical answer to the problem in hand. Stress is far more manageable if some plan of action has been agreed upon, or because the individual feels confident that they know what to do and have a belief in their ability to do it. Lipson and Lewitter-Koehler (1986) show that the sub-culture which develops around nurses continuously involved in high-stress psychiatry engenders mutual and self-support mechanisms. These in turn are often the product of a recognition by the nurses themselves that they are under stress. Such mechanisms are often informal, but provide the nurse with the confidence to practice.

Being able to predict changes in client needs, through careful observation and assessment; linking them with a predetermined personal or corporate nursing strategy, then putting the strategy into action with the knowledge that there are alternatives if things go wrong, seem to be crucial issues for nurses developing the skills for dealing with emergency situations, and particularly those of a psychiatric nature. These, and other, considerations will be dealt with in depth throughout the book, but it is important at this stage to establish just what is meant by a psychiatric emergency.

The psychiatric emergency

There are several definitions of emergency but all appear to have one thing in common, the necessity for immediate action. The word in general terms usually implies that something unforeseen has taken place, and certainly when used in a medical context, for instance within an Accident and Emergency Department, leaves people in little doubt that something extraordinary has taken place. The action required to deal with it is often seen as either specialist, or at least difficult. Certainly those who work for organizations which describe themselves as 'emergency services' see themselves as having to be prepared to do things which ordinary members of the general public would not be expected to do. However, the word is not often applied to situations which occur within a mental health setting. The term 'psychiatric emergency' (PE) is not widely used within the UK though in countries such as Germany, Holland and the USA it has specific meaning for all nurses. Unfortunately, the meaning differs depending on which country you practise in, and I suspect that UK nurses would have difficulty establishing a common understanding of it.

The American Psychiatric Association (1994) definition of a PE is, 'A situation that includes an acute disturbance in thought, behaviour, mood or social relationship that requires immediate intervention as defined by client, family or social unit'. Note, there is no mention of this occurring solely for mental health clients, nor any reference to the environment in which it may take place. The inference therefore, is that PE may take place within any clinical or non-clinical environment, with any client group and may not necessarily be dealt with by those specializing in mental health nursing. The problem with the APA definition is that it is cloaked in medical terminology, telling little of the actual presentation which might be expected. Fauman and Fauman (1981) extended this definition so that it gave some indication of the nature of the problem itself. They included:

1. behavioural alteration;
2. mood disturbance;
3. social relationship discordance;
4. thought disorder;
5. overwhelming nature of the problem;
6. prolonged or intense precipitant;
7. reduction in client's abilities and/or emotional strength at the time of the crisis.

However, this elaboration still does not clearly show what might be taking place. To appreciate fully the nature of an emergency it would seem necessary to explore what is happening to the individual who is experiencing it. All of us at certain times in our lives will feel desperate, frightened or angry, and these feelings may cause us to say and do things which ordinarily we would not. Certainly when having an argument with someone, especially when things do not seem to be going our way, we are prone to making statements which we regret later. It is difficult to say why we do such things, and even more difficult to say what we felt while we were saying them. The words seem to come of their own accord. It is almost as if we lose control of what we are saying, and in some extreme cases, what we are doing. Once this flashpoint has been reached there is no telling what can happen next. It would seem that the only thing which stops us from carrying out a totally violent or outrageous act is the sudden realization of what we are doing, and in some way we regain enough control to be able to restrict our actions to something a little more acceptable. In itself this momentary loss of control does not constitute an emergency, even though it may be both upsetting for those involved and cause concern and regret after the event. However, the more powerful the feelings we experience, and the less control we are able to exert over our responses, the greater the potential for a real emergency to occur.

In simple terms PE could be described as experiencing loss of control over one's actions resulting in behaviour that puts either the client or others at risk (Dang 1990). This lack of control usually requires the intervention of another person, in this case the nurse, to restore the behavioural balance and allow the client to resume control over his or her actions.

Soreff (1981) describes PE in terms of exhibited behaviour. He identifies four core elements which may be present:

1. change – and the client's response to it;
2. intolerance by the client – especially to change but also towards others involved in the situation;
3. the reaction of significant others – either towards the client, or as a response to the situation itself;
4. the immediacy of the situation – something has to be done right now.

The good point about this approach is that it sees PE as a continuum, enabling us to look back at what might have been the cause, and look forward to what might be done about it.

In the late 1940s when Caplan was developing his systems-based approach to a crisis-intervention framework he stated that the disturbance in a steady state of homeostasis was a common factor in the deterioration of an individual's ability to cope with stress (Caplan 1964). The only problem with using homeostasis as part of a PE definition is that it does not give credence to the psychopathology associated with such an event. It implies that psychological processes only occur as a result of an alteration in the individual's physical well-being. As we will see later, this may well be the case in situations where a client experiences physical pain, but most PEs develop as a direct response to the psychological processes themselves, tend to be more spontaneous than declining homeostatic stability would suggest and invariably incorporate emotional or perceptional disturbances.

Whichever approach is used to describe PE it is important to remember that there are always key components present. The client is going to say or do something which is dramatically different to, or a considerable exaggeration of, that which would normally be expected. This behaviour will probably result as a consequence of the client's intolerance to stress, and the cause of that stress may not necessarily be obvious to anyone else, and of course it may occur anywhere, and at any time.

Within the USA there is a wider appreciation among nurses that PE is not restricted to mental health environments alone, and this may be a reflection of the generic nature of their professional education programmes.

What it does show is a wider appreciation of the nurses' responsibility for mental health responses than that of traditionally specialist UK nurses. PE may happen within obvious places such as A&E departments, but it is just as likely to occur in midwifery settings, child care, doctors' or dentists' surgeries, general wards, out-patient clinics or community settings.

From a psychiatric nurse's point of view PE is more likely to occur within an acute admission setting, but of course may well happen anywhere that clients experience intolerable stress

Features of PE

There are no standard presentations for PE. A nurse confronted by a man threatening to jump down a stairwell in the centre of a busy general hospital will see a different picture to the nurse who has just been verbally abused by an apparently genteel elderly lady sitting in a quiet day hospital. However, some features are common to most emergencies.

1. The client is often extremely agitated or upset, and may be tearful and act in a highly distressed fashion.
2. Decisions made by the client at this time may be irrational and show very poor judgement.
3. Extreme demands are often made of others by those exhibiting these features.
4. The client may place himself or others in danger as a consequence of their behaviour.
5. The consequence of this danger is not usually obvious to the client.
6. Although not a necessary feature, but one which is sometimes present, the client may not be able to relate to the reality of his or her surroundings thus making statements which are difficult for others to deal with effectively.
7. Those having to deal with these features, and the effects they have upon the client's behaviour, may well feel frightened or distressed themselves, are then liable to respond spontaneously and are often left feeling hurt or angry after the event.

Causes of PE

While it is difficult to identify clearly what takes place during PE it is almost impossible to say why one should occur. The thoughts and feelings that an individual experiences in times of self-doubt, fear and desperation will depend very much on their own personal situation. Their perception of that situation will be determined by their own abilities to handle stress, and as a consequence may be totally different to that of another. To an observer the violent response of a client to a nurse's request for him to take some medication may seem completely out of context, but that is only because neither the observer, nor the nurse, have direct access to what is going on inside the client's head. A PE does not occur in a vacuum, and perhaps more importantly, the things that the client does at such times will seem appropriate to him, even though to the observer they may appear irrational and unacceptable. The client perceives a threat to their integrity and reacts accordingly, while the nurse asks a perfectly legitimate question and is struck in the face. Such is the difference in perception of the same event by the two participants. Who had the correct perception? Both of them, of course, but from their own personal understanding of what was taking place.

PE cannot always be considered simply as straightforward stimulus and response. Under normal circumstances if a nurse asks a client to have some medication the client will accept, but this is because the client understands why the request is being made, feels that the medication will do them good, does not feel threatened by the nurse, nor by the relationship which exists between them. However, what would happen if one or more of these elements were seen differently, say for example if the client felt that the medication was going to harm him, or if he considered that the nurse was threatening him in some way? Under such circumstances he might be expected to respond more aggressively. If indeed his beliefs were found to be correct then his behaviour would be considered appropriate.

If you were sitting in a railway station waiting for a train to arrive and all of a sudden someone came up behind you and tipped your chair backwards, then started to wheel you away from the waiting area, you would, to say the very least, become alarmed. If you were then deposited in a small white room, your clothes tampered with and the door slammed in your face leaving you imprisoned, your mental state would begin to deteriorate quite rapidly. When, after what seemed like an eternity in solitary confinement, someone returned, again tampered with your clothing, wheeled you out of the white room and back to the station waiting room, then left without any explanation, you would be entitled to be defensive, and subsequently even aggressive.

Such an event is not likely to happen, or is it? What if you were an elderly, confused and disoriented person, sitting quietly in the lounge of a hospital ward. Around you people are walking about, talking and quite busy. Music is playing in the background and your perception of this environment is that you must be in a railway station. A nurse decides to take you to the toilet, fails to tell you she is going to, wheels you there, leaves you for five minutes while she attends to someone else, returns and takes you back to the lounge. You lash out at her with clenched fists, shouting and kicking as you try to defend yourself against this personal attack. The nurse sees this as an unprovoked attack; you see it as a perfectly reasonable response to assault.

What caused the PE that resulted? Was it your mental state, which left you unable to make sense of your environment or the role and place of those within it correctly, or was it the nurse's intervention or her failure to communicate her intentions to you? Or was it the fear and indignity that was instilled inside you by the totally unacceptable sequence of events that took place?

Your response to the situation described above appears totally unacceptable when viewed from a purely observational standpoint, but seems understandable when analysed in more detail. Other situations may appear difficult to appreciate. If a client is refused permission to leave a clinical area, and therefore does not appear to be getting his own way, the verbal abuse which ensues could almost be seen as inevitable. Is it the situation which causes the PE, or is it the emotions that are generated in the client as a consequence of the situation? There are any number of different situations, each of which will be handled in a different way by the people involved, yet rarely will one of these situations develop into a PE. Therefore, it is the individual's perception of what is taking place, and the resultant feelings that they experience, which generate the potential for the PE, not the situation itself.

Of course, certain situations are more likely to precipitate PE than others, especially when a client perceives personal threat, or where actions taken by staff are in direct conflict with client needs or demands. Even in these situations it remains the psychological and emotional responses of those involved which will determine whether or not a PE occurs.

Nurses need to be aware of the psychological responses which might provoke PE if they are to be effective in diagnosing, intervening, and hopefully, avoiding, them. The main ones appear to be:

1. fear – accompanied by the sensation of helplessness, or linked in some way to self-preservation;
2. rejection – the feeling that of being totally alone and unwanted, without friends and of little consequence as an individual;
3. frustration – again associated with helplessness, and often as a direct result of being rejected, or feeling that no-one understands you or your needs;
4. intrusion – either physically into personal space, or psychologically into your thoughts and feelings, but always when uninvited or unwanted; this might also include an invasion of privacy;
5. inferiority – when others make you feel small or less important than you perceive yourself to be, possibly resulting in feeling that you are being taken advantage of;
6. embarrassment – as a result of failure, intrusion or feelings of inferiority;
7. grief – being inconsolable, and having others intrude upon your thoughts and feelings;
8. reality conflict – testing out the realness of a situation or relationship, and discovering weakness in yourself or others;
9. psychiatric disturbance – when mental health problems inhibit the ability to make proper sense of yourself or your surroundings, which in turn restrict judgement and effective problem tackling.

This last is particularly relevant to psychiatric nurses because it increases the unpredictability of client reactions and demands a greater awareness of their needs. For all nurses, the above represent a collection of indicators which need to be monitored carefully when trying to make sense of their client's responses.

Certain actions may exacerbate an imbalance of these indicators. For example, poor communication by either the client or the nurse; failure to explore the client's perceived needs; the nurse denying the possibility of intervention alternatives, or failing to recognize the individuality of each client; not involving the client in decision-making activities related to their own care; not establishing if there is a physical basis for the client's presentation (Waxman *et al.* 1984), or the failure to follow-up a client's care with adequate supervision once they have been discharged (Surles and McGurrin 1987). All of these may precipitate changes which the client finds stressful and difficult to cope with. In turn they may result in clients experiencing the irresistible feelings associated with indicators listed above, triggering a PE.

This last point is crucial to understanding the nature of PE. Just as in the situation where you are arguing with a friend over some minor issue, lose your temper, then self control, finally making outrageous statements which you later regret, so too the client experiencing PE may also be responding to an apparent minor point or situation. What is significant here is that the resultant behaviour is often uncontrollable, almost to the point of being irresistible. The nurse's controlled intervention at this time is a necessity if further harm is to be avoided.

High-risk clients

No client can be said to be totally immune from experiencing an emergency, but within a mental health environment certain client groups have been identified as being at risk more than others (Puskar and Obus 1989):

1. those who suffering from acute psychological disturbance – including panic attacks;
2. those suffering severe sadness;
3. those reacting to situational stress;
4. those undergoing detoxification programmes.

These are broad groupings, hence the terminology used to describe them, but they tend to be those clients most prone to reacting inappropriately, or in a desperate way, to what is going on around them.

Other clients are more at risk during different stages of their problem, hospitalization or treatment:

1. during admission;
2. during recovery from anaesthesia;
3. when medications are being changed;
4. when intoxicated;
5. when mental health problems are exacerbated by acute physical problems, including infections, constipation etc.

6. following a PE of another client;
7. prior to discharge;
8. while receiving follow-up care in a community setting;
9. those being cared for in an unfamiliar culture. Special attention must be paid to religious considerations.

PE and crisis intervention

Of course the actions or responses already discussed are often exhibited by clients in situations that would not be regarded as emergencies, but described as a 'crisis'. How is such an event defined, and does it differ from PE?

The literature often discusses PE under the heading of 'crisis intervention', but this is inaccurate. Crisis intervention is a specific approach to clinical action which differs from the immediacy associated with PE. Lego (1984) clearly shows that the difference between the two concepts is based upon outcomes, though this may be seen by some as a somewhat controversial point.

PE is described as an urgent situation which may occur repeatedly, requiring immediate action, but that this action will not necessarily bring about any real change in the client's life. Conversely, a crisis is often a turning point in a client's life which precludes the individual from carrying on as he or she has previously done. Lego is also at pains to point out that PE is limited to situations where the client is on the verge of total collapse or self-destructiveness, and emergency intervention is required to sustain life. A crisis may occur over a period of days, while an emergency appears to happen far more rapidly, perhaps taking just a few seconds from flashpoint to resumption.

The PE, therefore, differs from a crisis by both the immediacy of the required intervention, and its long-term effect upon the client.

One other key factor about PE is described by Soreff (1981), which perhaps highlights the difference between it, and crisis, best of all. In PE it is the patient who has the emergency, not the nurse, or the relative, or those standing watching. In a crisis, all those involved may be seen to be part of that crisis. In truth, when a client has an emergency, those standing by or attending usually suffer a crisis.

If one considers the primary aims of the nurse involved in PE, and there are two, these are also at variance with those of crisis intervention. These aims will be discussed in detail in Chapter 2, but briefly they are:

1. temporary stabilization – this may include stopping a client from running away, or from self harm, but will also involve the immediate release of the client's emotional tension;
2. cascade referral – in other words, referring the client on for further intervention once the emergency itself has been dealt with. This can be anything appropriate to the client's needs, and may also involve other disciplines or agencies.

By contrast, the long-standing goal of crisis intervention is to return the client to his or her pre-crisis level of functioning, or a higher one (Aquilera and Messick 1986). Crisis intervention, therefore, is not the same as PE. More significantly, any nurse might have to deal with PE, but specialist training is required for crisis intervention.

Research

As one might expect, the research covering issues of PE tend to be linked with that of crisis intervention, which in turn gives a misleading picture of both practice and resources (Geller 1991). However, that which deals specifically with PE is broadly based around the sub-groups of client groups (Ellison and Wharff 1985, Suokas and Lonnqvist 1989, Snowden and Holschuh 1992), interventions (Dunn 1989, Schmidt 1991), and services (Wellen *et al.* 1987, Corlito 1987). A fourth subgroup can be identified as being that which deals specifically with individual behavioural presentations which would, in themselves, be regarded as PE events, e.g. attempted suicide, violent incidents etc. (Porter-Tibberts 1986, Green 1988, Caplan 1993).

What is apparent from this literature is that those who are involved in the practice of PE nursing, say in an emergency department or an on-call group, regard themselves as specialist clinical practitioners. Those who have to deal with PE within the context of their daily work, and would therefore not regard this as one of their primary roles, see the process of PE nursing as a set of skills to be perfected by all nurses. Much the same dichotomy occurs when psychiatric nurses discuss the roles of counsellors and psychotherapists.

As they are with most current nursing practice issues, researchers are beginning to explore the nature and quality of PE nursing actions. For example, Schmidt (1991) developed an audit document which evaluated consistency of clinician's decision-making, and the resultant effects it had upon the client's progress following a PE incident, while Morgan (1989) looked at the effects clinicians might have upon the families of clients involved in PE. What these and other projects have in common is the necessity for nurses, and particularly those working in mental health, to not only understand the nature of PE but be able to have a series of options available to them should they be confronted with such an event. It may be possible that certain standard practices can be used during similar events and situations, but this has to be explained and researched before they can be regarded as correct, otherwise we may have situations where nurses use inappropriate nursing interventions which put both themselves and others at risk. Likewise, care which is effective at certain times needs to be explained so that nurses can make sense of what they are doing, selecting options on the basis of knowing what effects they will have, rather than choosing them because a reference book tells them to.

PE nursing research will tell the nurse a great deal about how to practise, but all those involved in PE must investigate their own, and their colleagues', performance during PE events if they are to develop the skills of dealing with them effectively.

Conclusion

An understanding of what constitutes a PE is essential if nurses are going to be effective in such situations. It is not enough to approach a violent incident with nothing more than a notion of getting it all sorted out, and nurses who prepare for such events always perform better during them as a consequence of their preparation. Professional practitioners are expected to provide effective interventions at all times and this can only be achieved if they have some understanding of what they are likely to have to deal with. Pusker and Obus (1989) indicate that staff must be able to make decisions under stress, tolerate ambiguity and realize that often there is no one correct choice to be made. This clinical objective will only be met when nurses have the correct information at their disposal; can differentiate between the necessity to do something immediately, or refer on at a later point in the event; appreciate something of what is happening to their client and know how to fit their intended interventions into the context of the client's personal requirements. Knowing what a PE is constitutes the first step in being able to deal with it.

References

American Psychiatric Association (1994). *Diagnostic and Statistical Manual of Mental Disorders*, 4th edn. APA, Washington DC.

Aquilera, D. and Messick, J. (1986). *Crisis Intervention: Theory and Methodology*, 5th edn. C. V. Mosby, St Louis.

Blomhoff, S., Seim, S. and Friis, S. (1990). Can prediction of violence among psychiatric inpatients be improved? *Hospital and Community Psychiatry*, 41(7): 771–75.

Cahill, C. D., Stuart, G. W., Laraia, M. T. and Arana, G. W. (1991). Inpatient management of violent behaviour: nursing prevention and intervention. *Issues in Mental Health Nursing*, 12:239–52.

Caplan, G. (1964). *Principles of Preventive Psychiatry*. Basic Books, New York.

Corlito, G., Martini, P., Domencic, F., Cesari, G. and Petrillo, M. (1987). A community alternative to psychiatric hospitalisation. *Mediterranean Journal of Social Psychiatry*, 11(1/2):69–79.

Dang, S. (1990). When the patient is out of control. *RN*, October, 57–8.

Dunn, J. (1989). Psychiatric intervention in the community hospital emergency room. *Journal of Nursing Administration* 19(10): 36–40

Ellison, J. M. and Wharff, E. A. (1985). More than a gateway: the role of the emergency psychiatric service in the community mental health network. *Hospital and Community Psychiatry*, 36: 180–85.

Fauman, B. J. and Fauman, M. A. (1981). *Emergency Psychiatry for the House Officer*. Williams & Wilkins, London.

Geller, J. L. (1991). 'Anyplace but the State Hospital': Examining assumptions about the benefits of Admission Diversion. *Hospital and Community Psychiatry*, 42(2): 145–52.

Gomez, R. (1983). Demographic and nondemographic characteristics of psychiatric emergency patients. *Psychiatric Clinics of North America*, 6:213–24.

Green, J. H. (1988). Frequent rehospitalisation and noncompliance with treatment. *Hospital and Community Psychiatry*, 39(9):963–6.

Lego, S. (1984). *The American Handbook of Psychiatric Nursing*. J. B. Lippincott Co., Philadelphia.

Lipson, J. and Koehler, S. L. (1986). The psychiatric emergency room: staff structure. *Issues in Mental Health Nursing*, 8:237–46.

Merker, M. S. (1986) Psychiatric emergency evaluation. *Nursing Clinics of North America*, 21(3):387–96.

Morgan, S. L. (1989). Families experience in psychiatric emergencies. *Hospital and Community Psychiatry*, 40(12):1265–9.

Porter-Tibberts, S. (1986). A compliance protocol: psychiatric emergencies and brief encounters. *Issues in Mental Health Nursing*, 8(3):223–36.

Pusker, K. P. and Obus, N. L. (1989). Management of the psychiatric emergency. *Nurse Practitioner*, 14(7):9–12, 14, 16, 18, 23, 26.

Rissmeyer, D. J. (1985). Crisis intervention alternatives in hospitalisation: why so few? *Psychosocial Rehabilitation Journal*, 9:54–63.

Schmidt, B. C. (1991). Clinical and economic influences on mental health triage decisions. Unpublished PhD thesis, University of Michigan, Michigan.

Snowden, L. R. and Holschuh, J. (1992). Ethnic differences in emergency care and hospitalisation in a programme for the severely mentally ill. *Community Mental Health Journal*, 28(4):281–91.

Soreff, S. M. (1981). *Management of the Psychiatric Emergency*, Wiley & Sons, New York.

Suokas, J. and Lonnqvist, L. (1989). Work stress has negative effects on the attitudes of emergency personnel towards patients who attempt suicide. *Acta Psychiatric Scandinavia*, 79:474–80.

Surles, R. and McGurrin, M. C. (1987). Increased use of psychiatric emergency services by young chronic mentally ill patients. *Hospital and Community Psychiatry*, 38(4):401–5.

Talley, S. and Chiverton, P. (1983). The psychiatric clinical specialist's impact on psychiatric emergency services. *General Hospital Psychiatry*, 5:242–5.

Waxman, H. M., Dubin, W., Klien, M., Weiss, K. J. and Carner, E. A. (1984). Geriatric psychiatry in the emergency department 2: Evaluation and treatment of geriatric and nongeriatric admissions. *Journal of the American Geriatrics Society*, 32(5):343–9.

Wellen, E., Slesinger, D. P. and Hollister, C. D. (1987). Psychiatric emergency services: evolution, adaptation and proliferation. *Sociology Science and Medicine*, **24**(6):475–82.

Suggested reading

Brownell, M-J. (1984). The concept of crisis: its utility for nursing. *Advances in Nursing Science*, July, 10–21. (Though titled as 'crisis' this paper deals with the problems associated with PE. Good background reading for establishing the differences between crisis intervention and PE.)

Brook, A. (1993). Emotional minefield. *Nursing Times*, **89**(3):48–9. (Short article looking at a client's ability to cope with physical illness and the effects such problems have upon her mental state.)

Ferry, R. (1992). Self-injurious behaviour. *Senior Nurse*, **12**(6):21–5. (Research project which explores SIB in Rampton Special Hospital, England. The conclusions made by the report show the necessity to establish the cause of any PE incident.)

McHaffie, H. E. (1992). Coping: an essential element of nursing. *Journal of Advanced Nursing*, 17:953–40. (Deals with many aspects of the professional coping process, giving an insight into the development of personal and clinical strategies.)

2

Psychiatric emergency nursing

Introduction

The indications are that, although there is always the potential for any person to have some form of emotional or personal crisis, only a small minority ever experience a full-blown psychiatric emergency. In the same way some nurses may go through the whole of their working careers and never have to deal with a client experiencing such an event, while others may have to do so far more regularly. In fact, PE is far more common than you might think, and as we have already seen not restricted solely to mental health settings. However, just as some clients are regarded as being at high risk of experiencing a PE, so some nurses work in areas where such events are far more likely to occur. Sometimes this is determined by the nature of the clinical environment, but more usually it is the client group, and the problems which they experience, which increases the possibility of PE work. Hence nurses working in emergency areas of any type, those who deal with extremes of physical or emotional presentations, and any that have to handle crisis situations, are most likely to be at the forefront of PE work.

By definition psychiatric nurses fall into this category. There are very few clinical areas which combine both the high-risk clients identified in Chapter 1 with the stress and emotional factors associated with PE in such a way as one might find in either in-patient or community mental health environments. Traditionally it is the acute areas which seem to have to deal with the more obvious examples of PE, but it is probably the case that a great many such incidents take place in the care of the elderly mentally ill, while community and rehabilitation staff will be only too familiar with situations which demand more extraordinary intervention than might be anticipated in such areas. The problem with determining how often such events take place is that very often they are not documented correctly, or are simply seen by the practitioners as part of the job. This causes not just problems in identifying the needs of the clients involved, but also creates difficulty for staff because they may not have had the opportunity to develop PE skills, which they are called upon to use quite regularly (Adler 1993).

If staff are not prepared correctly to identify when PE takes place, they will not be in a position to predict further events, take precautionary action or develop post-emergency strategies to reduce future risk. Such a situation is likely to produce poorer quality interventions and leave staff feeling threatened, abused and under-skilled. It is essential that all nurses make sense of their actions, and the effects they have upon their clients, and the very nature of potential or real PE situations makes it even more important that they have a clear under-standing of both their performance and potential for action. Any situation which is characterized by client anger, shock or panic, or generates concern about the safety of either the client or others has got to be seen as a probable PE. Recognizing this fact is the first step in preparing to develop an effective PE strategy (Merker 1986).

Psychiatric emergency nursing – what is it?

As we have already seen, PE nursing is having to deal effectively with high stress generated situations occurring at either end of an extreme behavioural continuum. A situation where a client is so depressed that they intend to take their own life is just as critical as one where the client is so over-active that they cannot recognize the danger in their attempt to use a bed sheet to hang glide from the roof of the hospital. Both clients present features of PE, yet are so markedly different in their behaviour. Significantly, however, both present the nurse with the same problem – what to do to save their lives.

PE nursing is bringing to bear the most effective care strategies at times of extreme crisis. It involves developing an operational policy which enables nurses to recognize the nature of the problems facing them, having a range of flexible alternatives to deal with them, evaluating their performance both during and after the event, and ensuring that follow-up procedures are instigated to support both themselves and the clients involved. If it is to work it has to be supervised and accurately documented so that staff are able to explore both the individual events as well as the nursing actions. It has to develop according to the range of PEs that occur and the suitability and effectiveness of the care offered. Finally, it has to take into account the context in which the event took place, recognize that PEs may last for as little as a few seconds, or as much as several hours, and that no matter how much planning takes place the nurses involved will not always make the right decisions, nor have the necessary resources (Murdach 1987).

While recognizing that there may be similarities between each PE event, or that certain clients behave in a similar fashion when experiencing high stress levels, the nurse must remember that each PE has to be tackled on its own merits. Whatever strategies are developed to deal with such events nurses must employ an individualized approach to the care they offer, with each client being seen as having a unique set of problems and responses. If nurses fail to adopt such an approach eventually their actions will become stereotyped, their effectiveness will be diluted by a lack of real awareness of the client's needs, and the intervention strategy will be a meaningless exercise. More importantly client contact at such times will become more threatening for the nurses and they will be more inclined to avoid PEs rather than do something about them.

PE nursing may involve three separate types of response:

1. verbal interventions;
2. physical interventions;
3. milieu management.

Nurses may use any one of these responses, or a combination of all of them. In most cases one form of intervention is usually more effective when reinforced by the use of another.

Two key factors need to be considered before any intervention is used within an emergency. Nurses need to take note of them before deciding upon either their operational policy or embarking upon individual responses to clients.

1. The client may be too angry, anxious or distressed to be able to respond appropriately to what is being said to them. They may not be able to follow directions, or appreciate the reassurances they are being offered.
2. It is probable that stress being experienced by the client is a result of some other underlying problem. It will be almost impossible for the nurse to deal with this other problem during the emergency, so it is of paramount importance to attend to the client's feelings and their immediate precipitants, rather than the deep-seated psychological trauma.

The aims of PE nursing

The primary function of any emergency intervention is to save life. However, while this might be the main purpose of the intervention in a psychiatric situation, the nurse's aim is more likely to be the reduction in emotional stress experienced by the client. It is important to differentiate between the subsequent outcomes of the intervention and the immediate effects it might have upon the client. It is the latter of these which constitutes the main purpose for carrying out PE nursing.

Certainly if a client were trying to cut his wrists with a piece of broken glass it would be vitally important to get the glass away from him. However, it might be far more important for the client if the feelings which inspired the action in the first place were dealt with so that he no longer felt the necessity to carry the action out. It would be the intensity of the client's emotional response which would be the main focus of the nurse's intervention, while at the same time being aware of the glass in his hand. Remember, it is the client who is experiencing the emergency, not the nurse.

Similarly, if a client was desperate to leave a clinical area against all medical and nursing advice, there might not be any immediate threat to his personal safety. However, his inability to make rational decisions about his actions or behaviour as a consequence of his intolerable levels of anxiety may require the nurse to intervene and stop him leaving. In doing so she would hope to help him to regain control of his feelings and construct a more positive personal strategy for dealing with his desire to leave hospital.

Of course, there are situations when the nature of the emergency is such that the main aim is definitely the preservation of life. If a nurse is attacked by a patient her first thought will inevitably be to ensure her own safety, while her second should be to work out how to resolve the client's feelings towards her so that he stops trying to hit her. As we will see throughout the book this can be achieved in a variety of ways, ranging from running to the nearest lockable room and shouting for help, to using break-away techniques and active listening (Urbaitis 1983).

However, the aims of PE nursing remain fundamental to its delivery and can be described as such:

1. to provide immediate support to a client suffering from the intense feelings associated with a PE;
2. to provide psychiatric first aid in the hope of reducing the emotional tension experienced by the client;
3. to protect both the client and the nurse from physical harm;
4. to help the client regain control of his feelings, and subsequently, his actions; if this is not possible because of the client's mental state, to help him regain enough composure to feel safe;
5. to help steer the client through the immediate feelings;
6. to be flexible and 'street-wise' in dealing individually with the client's needs;
7. reduce the impact of environmental factors which may be influencing the client;
8. get help or assistance where necessary;
9. evaluate the event both concurrently and retrospectively to determine how best to support the client during and after the event.

These aims have to be achieved as quickly and as effectively as possible. The key to the application of appropriate PE interventions is the knowledge of what to do, but it has to be done quickly, otherwise the situation could reach a point where it becomes totally out of control. Therefore, nurses must be brief in what they say, precise in what they do, practised in their technique, and safe in everything.

It is worth pointing out here that the aims of PE nursing do not include the development of detailed and on-going care plans after the event, nor in most cases post-event referral to other disciplines. As pointed out in Chapter 1 these are activities associated with crisis intervention and as such would complicate the intervening nurse's strategies for dealing with the immediacy of the situation. Should the same nurse be responsible for on-going care after the event this will be in the capacity of a key worker or primary nurse, not as the intervening nurse in an emergency situation.

What does PE nursing involve?

The details associated with various types of emergency interventions will be discussed in later chapters of this book. The purpose of this section is to outline the basis upon which a PE nursing strategy can be built. The elements described here are appropriate, whether or not they are to be used in developing a corporate strategy for a clinical area or group of nurses, or for one individual trying to improve her performance when confronted by an emergency.

Since the introduction of professional practices such as the nursing process, primary nursing and a more client-oriented approach to care, the ability of psychiatric nurses to prepare for, and ultimately deal with, PEs has been much improved. The nursing process in particular provides an ideal tool for providing an accurate baseline profile of individual clients, which in turn can help predict the potential crisis (Ward 1992). However, it is the way that the nursing process, and other contemporary practices, are incorporated into the overall care package which makes them effective.

There are several stages to developing a plan of action:

1. developing, where possible, an intimate knowledge of the client, his moods, feelings, pain and peace;

2. learning to use this information to predict the possibility for a PE;

3. intervening before a PE occurs, thus being able to be more objective in the way that the situation is dealt with, and reducing the client's possible embarrassment over his loss of control;

4. designing behavioural approaches which are known to have certain desired effects upon clients under stress;

5. identifying a system of support for nurses dealing with a PE;

6. practising the techniques to be used, either in role-play situations with other colleagues, or through contact analysis following previous PEs;

7. working out personal techniques for remaining as calm as possible during a PE situation;

8. exploring verbal and non-verbal approaches until individual nurses find those which they feel most confident about;

9. reading and researching PE strategies so that modifications and developments can be incorporated into the system;

10. keeping staff constantly aware of the operational protocols for dealing with PE, thus increasing their confidence and reducing the possibility of crisis avoidance;

11. ensuring that a post-emergency support system is in operation for nurses involved, so that reassurance can be provided and confidence boosted;

12. each incident to be carefully documented, giving specific details as to the nature of the whole event, not just what took place, or what was done.

In certain environments it may be possible to identify certain staff members who will deal with PE situations, although for many nurses, suddenly confronted by an abusive or disoriented client this may be impractical.

Of course, in many PE situations no amount of preparation will be able to overcome the feelings of fear or trepidation that the nurse experiences. Having a person standing right inside your personal space, shouting and spitting at you, is difficult for anyone to handle. Just because that person is a client and you are a nurse doesn't alter the feelings generated inside of you, except that you are supposed to do something positive about the incident. Nonetheless, knowing that there is a support system of other staff on their way to help you might restore the balance a little, but not a lot. You are still going to have to deal with this situation. Knowing that you have practised for this event in the past may instil slightly more confidence, and knowing that you have a series of personal skills that you can bring to bear should just be enough to help you get started. Manglass (1986) feels that most emergencies are manageable, with practice; it is only when the nurse loses control of herself and her own response to the client that real trouble starts. This may be true, but it is important that the nurse has confidence in her own abilities, those of her colleagues to support her in times of crisis, and the organization to support her after the event, which enable her to perform effectively in times of her own high stress (Chitty and Maynard 1986).

There are other factors which need to be incorporated into any strategy. These include the timing of clinical interventions. Sometimes it is not always necessary for the nurse to intervene directly a situation occurs. It may be far more important for a client to sort something out for himself, and if it is safe for him to do so the nurse may have to play a waiting role. In some situations one emergency may follow directly from another. At such times the nurse needs to know how to extricate the client from the proceedings to ensure his safety. Finally, knowledge of the emergency continuum, or the way that an emergency develops, its stages and final resumption, increases the nurse's awareness of what is happening, and hopefully reduces the apparent 'unknown' quality that is sometimes associated with such events.

Planning for a PE

Ultimately, the decisions that a nurse makes in any PE will be determined by their appreciation of the event, their ability to cope with stress and their personal confidence. However, one of the crucial components in any care strategy is the ability to plan what will happen when things step outside of the ordinary. Having alternatives is the nature of successful PE nursing. How can you plan for the extraordinary?

Morton (1986) feels that this is possible through careful observation, and certainly such a statement would appear to be supported by many other authors (Dubin *et al.* 1984, Butler 1987, Ward 1992, Daniels 1993). However, only a certain amount can be achieved using observational activities, and there are authors who feel that the subjectivity attributed to clinical client–nurse relationships may actually reduce the quality of data that is gathered (May 1991, 1993). What is important is that nurses gather information appropriate to the client's current situation, monitor the biopsychosocial effects that daily life has upon him, and compare this with the data they have about him. The observational material can only give an indication of what is taking place, and constantly needs updating.

However, planning for PE does not just mean that staff learn to predict client behaviours, it also means that they know exactly what they are going to do once one takes place. The outline strategy mentioned above only works if nurses produced it before an event takes place. The most effective care package is one which can deal with an emergency before it becomes one, the second best package is one which has the ability and planned resources to deal with any emergency once it has begun. If an emergency gets out of hand, it will be because either the staff were unprepared, or the resources necessary to contain it were unavailable, and also, therefore, unplanned.

Conclusion

Being able to nurse effectively during a psychiatric emergency is not something which just happens. Nurses have to gain experience, be properly prepared and supported and certain key components have to be considered before the experience to act as an efficient PE nurse is gained. The need to establish just how individual nurses function under stress, what their specific needs are, and how best to supervise them in their clinical practice have got to be seen as fundamentals to the development of any PE strategy.

Planning to work under stress can be just as important as actually doing it, while a generation of personal confidence and self-efficacy will only occur if nurses really do believe that those procedures and actions they have planned for will take place (Cavanagh and Snape 1993). Contemporary nursing practices have certainly helped psychiatric nurses. They have created a professional climate which credits client–nurse equality as the basis for care, and such a belief is central to the trust involved in developing the relationship between a client experiencing an emergency, and the nurse who is trying to help him deal with it.

The possibility that any nurse may be called upon to deal with a client who is having serious emotional problems is one that all psychiatric nurses face. Being able to predict that this problem may develop into any emergency is the first step in dealing with it; having the knowledge and skills to bring it to a positive conclusion should it develop further is the second stage. However, being able to make sense of it afterwards and do something to try to prevent it from happening again is the mark of an experienced PE nurse.

References

Adler, N. I. (1993). Analysis through work sampling of the role of the emergency nurse. *Journal of Emergency Nursing*, **19**(1):28–33.

Butler, J. P. (1987). Responding to the violent patient. *Nursing Life*, March/April:34–7.

Cavanagh, S. and Snape, J. (1993). Nurses under stress. *Senior Nurse*, **13**(2):40–2.

Chitty, K. K. and Maynard, C. K. (1986). Managing manipulation. *Journal of Psychosocial Nursing and Mental Health Services*, **24**(6):9–13.

Daniels, J. H. (1993). Believing the patient: the lost art of emergency nursing. *Journal of Emergency Nursing*, Guest Editorial, **19**(1).

Dubin, W. R., Hanke, N. and Nickens, H. W. (1984). *Psychiatric Emergencies*. Churchill Livingstone, New York.

Manglass, L. (1986). Psychiatric interventions you can use in an emergency. *RN*, **48**(11):38–9.

May, C. (1991). Affective neutrality and involvement in nurse–patient relationships: perceptions of appropriate behaviour among nurses in acute medical and surgical wards. *Journal of Advanced Nursing*, **16**:552–8.

May, C. (1993) Subjectivity and culpability in the constitution of nurse–patient relationships. *International Journal of Nursing Studies*, **30**(2):181–92.

Merker, M. S. (1986). Psychiatric emergency evaluation. *Nursing Clinics of North America*, 21(3):387–95.

Morton, P. G. (1986). Managing assault. *American Journal of Nursing*, 86(10):1114–16.

Murdach, A. D. (1987). Decision making in psychiatric emergencies. *Health and Social Work Journal*, 12(4):267–74.

Urbaitis, J. C. (1983). *Psychiatric Emergencies.* Appleton-Century-Crofts, Norwalk.

Ward, M. F. (1992). *The Nursing Process in Psychiatry*, 2nd edn. Churchill Livingstone, Edinburgh.

Suggested reading

Hoff, L. S. (1984) *People in Crisis: Understanding and Helping.* Addison-Wesley, California. (This work sets out the problems associated with people in crisis, drawing comparisons between crisis intervention and emergency psychiatry. It also looks at the role of practitioners and organizations for emergency care.)

Kupchik, D. (1985) Prevention and management of disturbed behaviour. *Canadian Journal of Psychiatric Nursing*, 26(4):9–11. (Though only dealing with one aspect of emergency the concept of prevention in this article is relevant to most emergency situations. Good analysis of individual intervention techniques.)

Lowe, T. (1992). Characteristics of effective nursing interventions in the management of challenging behaviour. *Journal of Advanced Nursing*, 17:1226–32. (This research report identifies 10 characteristics which are seen as intervention effective, and explores them within a clinical management setting.)

Pusker, K. R. and Obus, N. L. (1989). Management of the psychiatric emergency. *Nurse Practitioner*, 14(7): 9–12, 14, 16. (This article is something of a classic. It gives very in depth analysis of the psychiatric emergency and outlines a whole range of practical alternatives for setting up PE nursing packages.)

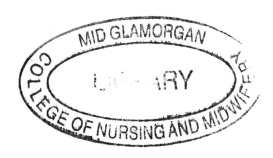

3

Professional coping strategies

Introduction

Chapter 1 began by asking a series of questions about our ability to deal with difficult or embarrassing situations. It concluded that all of us eventually cope in some way with most things in our lives. This is also true of professional nurses. It would seem that no matter what they are asked to do they always appear to be able to find a way of doing it. At work most people have a range of 'things' that they might ordinarily expect to happen, some that could happen, and a couple more that shouldn't, but on rare occasions, do happen. The first two of these groups usually require the implementation of a set of procedures or protocols to be able to deal with them. The third group, in most cases though not too serious, still causes confusion and possibly alarm, but will eventually be sorted out.

Because nurses deal with people's lives and their well being it stands to reason that the procedures and protocols used to deal with the first two groups will be well covered in the nurse's education and professional development. Skill will be required to implement them, but at least the nurse will have guidelines as to what is needed. However, the methods used to deal with the third group will depend largely upon the personal resources of the individual nurse, and are likely to be further complicated by the extreme nature of the situation, i.e. life-threatening, and the fact that the nurse may be totally responsible for what happens. An emergency situation at the checkout of a supermarket, when a customer is angered by the behaviour of the staff, does not contain the same level of danger as one associated with a client attempting to take his own life, even though the first of these may possibly lead to the second. In other words the nature of the third group, or as they should be called, emergencies, is far more stressful for nurses than for many other groups of workers. The person on the checkout can choose to ignore the customer, call for assistance or simply apologize. The incident is over and done with and, perhaps with the exception of some hurt pride, can be forgotten. The nurse cannot ignore the client, may be totally unsupported, and will need to summon more personal skill than a simple apology if the client is to be prevented from harming him/herself. While such an example is not intended to demean the work of those working at supermarket checkouts it does illustrate the main difference between the two occupations, the level of responsibility and associated stress attributed to being a nurse (Handy 1991).

The question which has to be asked at the beginning of this chapter is one which has been posed by many authors in recent years (Hiscott and Conrop 1989, McGrath *et al.* 1989, Schaefer and Peterson 1992). Are nurses, and in particular mental health nurses, so well prepared that they are able to cope with every eventuality, and in particular emergencies? Because, as Way *et al.* (1992) and Thomas (1993) indicate the nature of psychiatric care is changing, and the incidence of group three incidents, as described above, is becoming more regular (Guze and Unutzer 1993).

What does 'coping' mean?

Coping means different things to different people. For many it is simply 'getting by', while others would view it as 'resolving problems' or 'finding solutions'. In effect it means different things to different people depending upon their expectations, previous experience and self-confidence. It is also dependent upon the nature of the problem, the environment in which it occurs, the perception of its importance by those involved in its resolution, and the degree of control the individual has, both over the problem and those affected by it. All of these factors will influence the individual's ability to cope at a given time; thus on one day major difficulties can be dealt with clearly and confidently, yet the next day even the smallest of problems appears insurmountable. Coping has to be seen as something which changes in relation to the factors described above and not something which once achieved can be replicated automatically. Some people are identified as those who cope, others as those who do not. This, however, is both too simplistic a view as well as probably being untrue. Some people's capacity for coping may be more refined by experience and personal confidence than others, but all have the ability to cope. It is the nature of their coping styles which differentiates them from one another.

Most models of coping recognize the importance of maintaining a balance between, on the one hand, being able to solve problems, and on the other, being able to adapt to the consequences of not being able to solve them. In simple terms coping is about dealing with stress. A certain amount of stress can induce an individual to work harder and more efficiently by arousing and alerting them, and can therefore be quite a healthy thing. However, higher levels of stress are uncomfortable and begin to interfere with the individual's ability to maintain the balance between excitement and peace of mind. As the level of stress is increased, so the individual's performance may become affected, eventually reducing it to inefficiency. If the level of stress continues to rise beyond the individual's personal threshold they may not be able to do anything at all. The resultant frustration may produce feelings of anger, resentment and isolation which can be directed either outwardly, at those seen as responsible for the situation, or inwardly, towards the individual him/herself. Either way the result is of feelings of failure which may have serious consequences for those involved. Ultimately the emotional cost to the individual may result in the need to seek professional help, or, in our society, it may be thrust upon them as a result of his actions towards himself or others.

Using this model, coping would be regarded as the point at which an optimum performance was attained in relation to the amount of stress being experienced. Conversely, not coping would be the point at which performance was ineffective in the presence of stress (Gross 1992). However, as McHaffie (1992) points out when describing the phenomenological transactional coping model of Lazarus and Folkman (1984), nothing is really that simple! Too many factors need to be considered to be able to reduce the process of coping to a point where it can be defined without reference to those factors. Nevertheless, the one constant factor in any model of coping is its relationship to stress.

The stress factor

Stress is measured, albeit subjectively, by the amount of anxiety that it generates. We have two alternatives when confronted by this anxiety. We can either deal with the problem which confronts us, and literally remove the anxiety, or we can deal with the feelings of anxiety without dealing with the problem. The first of these is considered to be direct coping, the second, indirect, or avoidance coping. The action we take to initiate either of these two approaches is referred to as coping behaviours.

For example, if a nurse is experiencing difficulty working with a particular client, and this has led to friction between the two of them, the stress levels of the nurse will probably rise. Anxiety will be experienced whenever contact with the client is expected or occurs. This in turn will have a direct bearing on the quality of the nurse's interventions and subsequently the client's attitude towards the care environment. The whole situation may escalate into either total therapeutic inactivity or a violent outburst. The problem for the nurse is the difficulty experienced in making decisions about what to do, while the result is the anxiety this indecision provokes. If direct coping is used, the nurse will discuss the situation with a clinical supervisor, colleague and probably the client, develop an alternative strategy and put it into operation. The result would probably be a reduction in the anxiety level because the inactivity had been dealt with.

Alternatively, if indirect coping is used, the nurse would avoid contact with the client and resist attempts by colleagues to discuss the situation. The result would probably be a considerable reduction in perceived anxiety because the inactivity did not need to be dealt with. However, the consequence of this action would be to reduce both client and nurse confidence. Eventually the nurse would be required to re-establish contact with the client, or account for her lack of action. Without the benefit of previous problem-solving experience to fall back on it is likely that she would perform very ineffectively, and by default, experience the return of the anxiety.

While it can be seen from this example that direct coping is probably the most effective way of dealing with anxiety, it is not always an option open to us. Things have to be done as and when they can and sometimes responses to problems must be delayed because of other things that are happening. Also, direct coping can be anxiety-provoking in itself and this may be a deterrent in some situations. A balance between direct and indirect coping has to be achieved. The model discussed here is a derivation of that described by Hans Selye (1956). By necessity, it is a simplistic one used for the purpose of developing practical strategies later in the book. The reader is urged to explore alternative coping mechanisms in an attempt to find one which best suits their personal style. Some examples are provided in the suggested reading section at the end of this chapter.

Stress factors in psychiatric nursing

In recent years several researchers have attempted to explore the nature of stress factors for mental health and psychiatric nurses within their professional environment (Trygstad 1986, Jones *et al.* 1987, Snibbe *et al.* 1989, Sullivan 1993). Examination of their work reveals that the stressors come under three main headings: those related to the client group, those related to the working environment and those related to the relationships that develop between the nurse and other professionals, including other nurses.

Sullivan points out that it is usually assumed psychiatric nursing is stressful, and perhaps the natural assumption to make from that is, that it is the nature of the client group, and contact with them, which make it so. What is interesting about these, and other studies, however, is just how low on the stressor scale client contact is rated, in contrast to contact with peers and nursing seniors which is often seen as very stressful. Jones describes the 'demands of the job', while Trygstad indicated that it was not so much the client who generated the stress, as the nurse's perception of what might happen if the client did not respond favourably to the nurse's actions. This seems to suggest that it was the nurse questioning her own ability, coupled with the affects of a lively imagination, which generated high stress levels. This again is interesting because, as we will see later, many nurses feel that their best source of help when confronted by an emergency is their own behaviour. However, it would be wrong to deduce from this research that nurses only have to deal with stress in any one of these three areas at any one time. In many cases it is as a result of a culmination of stresses that a particular coping dilemma arises.

For example, on one day the nurse may be working with other members of staff with whom she gets on well. They understand each other, have similar ways of doing things and trust in each other's judgement and skills. They provide each other with support and guidance when needed and generally work well as a team. If an emergency occurs on such a day the likelihood is that there will be a collective response to it, with each member of staff supporting the other. The nurse will not feel stranded between her own decisions and the consequences of her actions. The effect on her confidence will be to strengthen her belief in her own capabilities and possibly deal more effectively as an individual practitioner, safe in the knowledge that she is not on her own.

Take the same situation or emergency and place it in the same clinical area on another day. Here we find the same nurse, who coped well under the previous set of circumstances, but working with a different group of nurses. She does not know them very well, and there appears to be divisions among them about roles and responsibilities. They do not appear to get on well together, disagree about clinical options for their clients, resent supervision and are at odds with nurse management about staffing levels and off-duty rotas. Each one feels that they have the correct answer to problems that might otherwise be seen as requiring joint answers. Their collective confidence as a team is low and their support for each other is minimal. Under these circumstances the nurse performs badly. Not only does she feel unsupported, but in practice she is left to her own devices, knowing that eventually she may well be criticized for any approach she adopts. Her stress levels are already much higher than on the previous day, even before the emergency occurs, and the consequence is that she does not respond to it in the same way as before. Oh, she may think that she is doing the same thing, but it is the quality of the responses that is different, and the confidence with which she acts, that has changed.

Thus, the nurse who was quite able to cope one day, was unable to cope the next, even though the perceived problem was the same. The difference lay in her feelings about herself in relation to those with whom she was working. Such situations are not uncommon within caring professions. The very nature of nursing itself and the process of caring generates high stress factors that are not necessarily found in other occupations. The psychiatric client group, with its inherent behavioural instability, cannot be attributed as being the only stress factor, otherwise it would be easy to regulate for their behavioural demands and irregularities. If this were possible eventually there would be no such thing as a psychiatric emergency because everyone would know how to deal with it. This is, however, obviously not the case. It is the interplay of other stress factors within the workplace, and within the nurse's personal life that determine their ability to take on board, and deal effectively with, the added stress generated by the psychiatric emergency. It is necessary for nurses to be aware of such stressors, to appreciate how they affect their performance and to be positive in their approaches to dealing with them.

The stressor groups indicated by nurse researchers can only begin to tell us what is happening to nurses within the workplace. It cannot tell us what is happening inside a nurse's head when things go wrong, when the client abuses the nurse, when demands are made that threaten the self-esteem and dignity of the nurse, or when the feelings of failure well up and the nurse has no-one to turn to for help. What it can do is start the process of realization that all nurses face the same types of problems and that if they have some understanding of how they develop and what is happening they have a better chance of being able to deal effectively with them. What the research into stressors, the models of coping and the theories of response tell us is that nurses cannot be expected to deal with emergencies on their own. They cannot be held responsible for dealing with all the stressors, just as they cannot be held accountable for resolving the interpersonal differences that may exist within a clinical team, or the quality of the furnishings in a ward, or the lack of suitable accommodation for clients within the community. But, they do have to remember that if these things affect them, then they are certainly going to affect their clients.

Coping strategies for the client group

Just as nurses are subject to a series of external stressors, so too is their client group. The work of Weaver *et al.* (1978), Caseem (1984) and Pearson *et al.* (1986) shows that those with mental health problems have a variety of coping mechanisms for dealing with stress, but that the stress itself is often generated by an unusual collection of factors. As one might expect frustration at clinical and personal events would appear to be high on the list of factors, with the affect and consequences of psychological difficulties also rating quite highly, but so do disagreements about food and personal space, jealousy issues and relationship problems. The main difference between the nurse and the client, when considering responses to stress, is that the nurse is usually a member of a team, whereas the client is usually on their own, both physically and psychologically. In most cases the client's coping strategies are limited, not only because of those psychological difficulties but other things such as the lack of privacy, freedom of movement and access to external sources of stress reduction, such as recreational activities or socializing with friends. Such limitations are likely to provoke more strenuous responses to stress, because there are so few alternatives open to the client for dealing with it.

In many cases the clients' dependence on avoidance coping strategies may well have been a precursor to the psychological difficulties they experience. Their apparent lack of power within the client–nurse relationship, and the perceived dominance of the nurse may also contribute to their frustration. We must also consider what role medications, and the client's willingness to take them, have within this relationship, and what effects they may have upon the stress levels of those clients (Pearson *et al.* 1986). For, as we have seen already, many of the beliefs we have about what happens between clients and nurses, when tested, prove to be false. It may well be that in some cases the therapeutic effects of medication may be outweighed by the stress the client feels in having to take them.

Self-awareness

Just as it is important for us to explore reasons why clients both experience and respond to stress in the way that they do, it is also important that nurses are aware of the effects of stress upon themselves. By this I do not mean the making of narrow-minded and totally useless statements such as, 'I sometimes feel a little stressed out at work, but I don't let it get through to me.' Such a lack of insight, and an almost childlike dependence upon superficiality as an explanation for complex interpersonal behaviours, is both time-wasting and potentially dangerous. If nurses cannot make accurate assessments about what is happening to them, and why, how can they expect to do the same in relation to their clients? If they are unable to assess the client's needs, how will they be able to decide what strategy or personal skill to use to facilitate their satisfaction? Indeed, how will they even know what personal skills they have?

It is imperative that nurses find out which stressors they have the most difficulty working through, and what sort of techniques they use to overcome them. Equally so they must identify how this stress affects their behaviour, and what others say about them when they appear to be working under stress. They need to explore the possibility that some stressors are just too difficult to tackle head-on and need to be considered from a distance before being dealt with. They have to observe the actions of others and relate it back to their own experiences. They have to be honest about their capabilities, and seek the advice of supervisors in deciding what to do about their performance. They have to explore the nature of their own needs, and recognize that there is a big difference between what they really need, what they think they need and what they want.

The key here is the truthfulness with which the subject is approached. To be able to develop as a practitioner, the nurse has to know what they are starting off with in the first place. Once this has been established then it is possible to explore personal alternatives which would otherwise have remained undiscovered.

Becoming self-aware is not, however, a process which should be carried out on your own. Certainly a great deal of the work is personal and intimate, therefore potentially painful, but that doesn't mean that you have to put yourself into solitary confinement. Perhaps the hardest part about self-awareness is coming to terms with feelings of inadequacy, or simply the realization that you find it difficult to cope at certain times. For this reason it is important that you have someone who is prepared to listen to what you have to say, and provide encouragement and support for you while you seek either to accommodate this new found information into your perception of yourself, or work towards using it for change. Whatever is decided, this too has to be discussed and assimilated. Self-awareness is not self-denial. It has to be something which gives the individual a greater understanding about they way he/she behaves, and subsequently provides the basis for an increase in their personal skills and professional effectiveness (Bond 1986).

Of course the other reason for having some sort of mentor while trying to make sense of your behaviour is that the other person is in a position to show you that you are not the only one who behaves, feels and responds the way you do. Part of the reason why people do not disclose information about themselves is that they feel they are the only one who does what they do! Being told that this is not the case can often be a tremendous relief in itself. Sharing experiences and trying to resolve conflict and stressor behaviour with either a friend or close working colleague can admittedly sound threatening, but the vast majority of nurses who attempt it find that it is nowhere near as stressful as they believe it to be (Burnard 1990).

Self-awareness is not just an exercise in mutual support and personal development. It reflects an intention on the part of the nurse to be effective within the professional arena, and to assume the responsibilities of providing appropriate interventions, irrespective of the circumstances in which they are required. Although it is possible to detect changes in client behaviour, and intervene effectively before things get out of control, emergency situations may still occur and will require spontaneous and imaginative responses. These can only be provided by a nurse who has thought the problem through beforehand; has considered what to do, and how; has planned for this eventuality long before it happened, but above all else believes that they are capable of resolving the emergency in a positive manner. Certainly some nurses will appear to work instinctively, will seem to know just what to do without apparently thinking about it. Don't be fooled! They thought about, or did it before, and then thought about it again, analysed it and stored their decisions away for the next occasion when they would be needed.

The purpose of preparation

We have seen that it is possible to deal effectively with stress and, as a consequence, perform with a degree of confidence, thus increasing the potential for successful intervention during an emergency. However, preparation is not just about being self aware, though it is certainly a key issue. There is little point in knowing how you perform under stress, if when you experience it you do not carry out the self-awareness routines that have given you your personal baseline in the first place. Self-awareness is, after all, just a response to a set of variables. You may know that you will behave in a certain way when

- someone else is present;
- you feel supported;
- you know the client concerned; and
- you feel wide awake and alert.

Each time an emergency occurs and these variables are present, you will behave as you anticipated. But, although variables cannot change, they can be influenced by other variables. They are only the circumstances in which an event takes place. If

- no-one else is present;
- you do not feel supported;

- you do not know the client; and
- you were up half the night looking after your sick pet dog,

then you are not going to behave the way you thought you would. You only need to change one variable and reassessment becomes necessary. The reality is that you cannot predict the way you will behave in any situation. All you can hope to do is give yourself some indication of the range of behaviours that are available; which ones you are good at, and which ones you are not.

So, preparation is about having some degree of understanding about what you can do, and having the resources to be able to do it. Invariably when nurses respond to an emergency situation there are likely to be other people in the vicinity. They do not have to be other nurses, or even health-care professionals, just someone who is there. Part of the sensation of confidence comes from knowing that if you are in some sort of trouble there is someone there to help you out. However, if you have never discussed with them what it is you are going to do, then they will have no real idea of how to support you. Therefore, the final component of preparation is discussing with your colleagues what you intend to do and what might happen as a consequence. Colleagues could mean other nurses, but it might mean a client's family or friends, especially if you are working within a community setting, or it might mean other professionals, such as teachers or social workers. Whoever they may be, planning, based on assessed knowledge of self and others, and discussed in full with those involved, is the key to preparation.

Personal technology and self-doubt

What happens when you are asked to deal with an emergency will largely depend on the variables we have already discussed. Everything, from the way you feel about yourself, to the way the client perceives what you are attempting to do, will have some part to play. The one issue we have not covered are the skills that will be required to deal with the emergency. In the next chapter we will be looking at strategies that can be adopted, but it is the personal skill of the individual nurse which will enable them to put those strategies into practice, and it is the confidence that the nurse has in herself which enables her to use those skills. Skills, or personal technology, are the techniques and behaviours that the nurse has developed to link her with her clients. They are the methods through which she uses the strength of her own personality to support those of her clients. But, just as the client needs the confidence to use the skills learnt during therapy to deal with their pain and their peace, so too does the nurse need the confidence to use her personal technology. Without it she will never explore the behaviours of change and development, will never challenge her own resources nor dare to attempt things for the first time, or take chances, be successful, or fail and try again.

In an emergency situation there will very often be little time to think about what comes next. When a nurse is confronted by overwhelming odds, or the danger is far too great, then that nurse has every right to run away. He/she may run to the next clinical area, or shout for help from inside a locked lavatory, but either way running away is the right decision to make. What is important is not so much that the nurse got away, but what they do afterwards – i.e. seeking help to deal with the emergency. The nurse did not just leave the problem for someone else to find, they coped using the safest method available at the time. This is a great deal different to seeing a dangerous situation develop and just walking away, pretending that you knew nothing about it, or allowing others to deal with it without providing any support or back-up.

Running away from an emergency may be the most sensible thing to do if you cannot deal with it yourself, but running to summon support is the act of a professional, taking responsibility for getting things done. Sometimes it takes a tremendous amount of personal courage, a fact often overlooked by nurse managers, the media and the general public, but more important than that, it takes confidence in oneself to be able to do it. Confidence to be able to make a decision and see it through. Confidence to be able to make yourself the centre of attraction in an attempt to summon assistance. Confidence not to give in, and confidence to take the responsibility required to resolve the situation.

Pretending that you knew nothing of a situation before it occurred, or failing to support colleagues when things become dangerous, is to some degree understandable, especially if you are very frightened, but within a nursing context, it is unacceptable. Nurses who do not respond to the challenge of accountability become a liability. Nurses have to support each other, have to be prepared to listen to each others' needs, then plan the systems that will provide them with the confidence to use them. They have to trust in the abilities of each other and they have to believe that when difficult times arrive they will not be left unsupported. These are fundamental team qualities that must be present if psychiatric emergencies are, in the first instance to be avoided, and in the event of their taking place, dealt with in the most positive and effective way. There is no point in discussing the strategies in Chapter 4 if the nurse has not first explored their responses to stress, taken the time to consider the needs of those with whom they work and discussed issues related to support and supervision. Then, and only then, is it possible to look at the uses to which the confident application of personal technology can be made.

Conclusion

Have we answered the question posed at the beginning of the chapter? Are nurses properly prepared to deal with any emergency? Well, only the individual nurse will know if that is true, but if they answer 'yes', it will be because they have already considered the main points of the chapter. We have explored the duality of stress, and responses to it. Duality, yes, because isn't it strange that nurses have to deal with psychiatric emergencies, which in themselves are invariably caused because of increases in client stress, yet nurses are expected to be able to deal with their own experience of stress at such times?

The expectations of nurses, especially those dealing with areas of human behaviour that the general public finds it difficult to cope with under any circumstances, remain very great. Nurses' coping qualities have reached almost mythical status, but this is truly an enigma, for no matter how ever-present nursing interventions are during times of conflict and crisis, the fact remains that nurses have to learn how to deal effectively with them. The sad thing is that some never do. Intuition, whatever that is, has very little to do with it. Assessing, planning and evaluating are the main corporate ingredients, while self-awareness; self-confidence and personal technology form the basis of the individual's input. In the next chapter we deal with the strategies that can be developed once these crucial variables have been considered.

References

Bond, M. (1986). *Stress and Self-awareness: A Guide for Nurses.* Butterworth-Heinemann, Oxford.

Burnard, P. (1990). *Learning Human Skills: An Experiential Guide for Nurses*, 2nd edn. Butterworth-Heinemann, Oxford.

Caseem, M. (1984). Violence on the wards. *Nursing Mirror*, **158**(21):14–16.

Gross, R. D. (1992). Motivation, emotion and stress. Chapter 6 in *Psychology – The Science of Mind and Behaviour*, 2nd edn. Hodder & Stoughton, Sevenoaks.

Guze, B. H. and Unutzer, J. (1993). Studies of psychiatric inpatients. *Current Opinion in Psychiatry*, **6**(2):233–7.

Handy, J. A. (1991). The social context of occupational stress a caring profession. *Social Science and Medicine*, **32**(7):819–30.

Hiscott, R. D. and Conrop, P. J. (1989) Job stress and occupational differences among mental health professionals. *Sociology and Social Research*, **74**(1):10–15.

Jones, J. G., Janman, K., Payne, R. L. and Rick, J. T. (1987). Some determinants of stress in psychiatric nurses. *International Journal of Nursing Studies*, **24**(2):129–44.

Lazarus, R. S. and Folkman, S. (1984). *Stress: Appraisal and Coping.* Springer, New York.

McGrath, A., Reid, N. and Boone, J. (1989). Occupational stress in nursing. *International Journal of Nursing Studies*, **28**(4):343–58.

McHaffie, H. E. (1992). Coping: an essential element of nursing. *Journal of Advanced Nursing*, **17**:933–40.

Pearson, M., Wilmot, E. and Padi, M. (1986). A study of violent behaviour amoungst in-patients in a psychiatric hospital. *British Journal of Psychiatry*, **149**:232–5.

Schaefer, K. M. and Peterson, K. (1992). Effectiveness of coping strategies among critical care nurses. *Dimensions of Critical Care Nursing*, **11**(1):28–34.

Selye, H. (1956). *The Stress of Life*, McGraw-Hill, USA

Snibbe, J. R., Radcliffe, T., Weisberger, C., Richards, M. and Kelly, J. (1989). Burnout among primary care physicians and mental health professionals in a managed care setting. *Psychological Reports*, **65**:775–80.

Sullivan, P. J. (1993). Occupational stress in psychiatric nursing. *Journal of Advanced Nursing*, **18**:591–601.

Thomas, B. (1993). Nurses must adapt to changes in hospital care. *British Journal of Nursing*. 2(14):698–9.

Trygstad, L. N. (1986). Stress and coping in psychiatric nursing. *Journal of Psychosocial Nursing and Mental Health Services*, **24**(10):23–7.

Way, B. B., Evans, M. E. and Banks, S. M. (1992). Factors predicting referral to inpatient or outpatient treatment from psychiatric emergency services. *Hospital and Community Psychiatry*, **43**:703–8.

Weaver, S. M., Brooke, A. K. and Kat, B. J. B. (1978). Some patterns of disturbed behaviour in a closed ward environment. *Journal of Advanced Nursing*, **3**:251–63.

Suggested reading

Brooks, N. and McKinlay, W. W. (1992). Mental health consequences of the Lockerbie disaster. *Journal of Traumatic Stress*, Oct., **5**(4):527–43. (While this relates directly to the mental health of those involved in a major disaster, there are lessons to be learnt about stress responses generally.)

Robinson, S. E., Roth, S. L., Keim, J., Levenson, M. *et al.* (1991). Nurse burnout: work related and demographic factors as culprits. *Research in Nursing and Health*, **14**(3):223–8. (Good study exploring a wide range of factors which impact upon nurse performance, self-efficacy and clinical effectiveness.)

Wykes, T. and Whittington, R. (1991). Coping strategies used by staff following assault: an exploratory study. *Work and Stress*, Jan.–Mar., **5**(1):37–48. (The authors consider staff responses to personal assault. They offer a series of alternatives but highlight the difficulties some staff have in coming to terms with the event, and its consequences for clinical practice.)

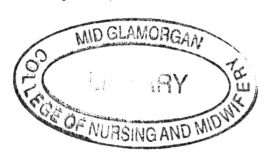

4

Intervention principles

Introduction

Having considered the nature of the psychiatric emergency, the main problems facing those who have to deal with them, and some of the strategies used to cope with the stress generated by such events, the next step is to look at the types of interventions that might be of value when the nurse is faced by a PE.

There is always some sort of 'general rule' that applies to all intervention techniques, and tackling a PE is no different. We will explore some basic principles and then expand upon them to consider how they might be developed, and what the alternatives are. The keyword for this chapter is 'adaptability'. No matter how much reading an individual does, and no matter what alternatives and creative approaches may have been considered, when a PE occurs these will only be guidelines. For each PE will pose new problems, and each set of circumstances will suggest their own variations upon the chosen clinical action. The nurse has to be adaptable, because it is not possible to make an emergency situation fit the technique that the nurse wants to use for it; the nurse has to use the techniques which best suit the emergency.

Historically this has not always been the case. Clients who confronted staff, or even questioned the organization's rules, have been faced with very aggressive and strong handed responses (Weaver *et al.* 1978). Certainly in mental health settings, where most of the staff were male, and chosen for the profession on the basis of their physical prowess rather than their caring attitude, the use of restraints and seclusion were nearly always preceded by some sort of rough handling (Norris and Kennedy 1992). Clients could guarantee that if they were involved in an emergency, it would be dealt with swiftly, and in some cases quite painfully. Unfortunately, the problems which caused the emergency would not be dealt with, and the whole intention of the nurses' actions would be to restore order to the clinical area. Many clients were simply jumped upon by over-zealous nurses, and left behind locked doors until they calmed down. Fortunately in the UK this is no longer an acceptable option. The social climate and political agenda have combined to ensure that clients' rights have become the driving force for care developments. This has meant that not only are there structures in place which dictate how care should be organized, but individual nurses have to ensure that the personal interventions they offer are based primarily upon the demands of the client group.

Where does the nurse gain the experience to deal with an emergency? It is probably only through experience of such events that the nurses learn to explore the use of alternative approaches, but such exploration has to begin the very first time that such an event takes place. The supervision and support offered to beginning nurses may often be the main determinant in the way that they develop as practitioners for the rest of their careers. However, every nurse has to start somewhere.

The game plan (AIRS)

The game plan is a rough outline of what it is you intend to do. In a sporting sense, it means how do you intend to play the game, or what is your strategy for winning a bout? The idea behind a game plan is that it gives you a starting point, gives you a certain amount of confidence in your ability to cope, and you do not have to think too much at the time of crisis about what to do next, because you already have a plan. It provides you with the basis upon which you can build more detailed and effective strategies.

In the case of a PE it means what you can do to get the most positive result. The PE game plan has four main components:

1. assessment,
2. intervention,
3. resolution,
4. support.

These four (AIRS) will be discussed in detail later in the chapter, but it would be useful to explore what they mean before progressing. Consider this example.

> Robert has been on the ward for several days. He was admitted onto a drug detoxification programme and is experiencing severe psychological and physical withdrawal problems. He desperately wants something to help him overcome the symptoms he is experiencing, but Karen, his primary nurse, is not prepared to override the programme protocols which prohibit additional medication. Robert is becoming increasingly agitated, pacing up and down and shouting that no-one cares what happens to him. He has already threatened to leave the ward if he does not get help soon, and has given Karen an ultimatum. He will leave if the doctor has not seen him within the next ten minutes.

Karen explains that this is not possible, and Robert rushes forward towards her, reaching out to grab hold of her. She responds by moving backwards, and to one side, and Robert, already unsteady on his feet, collides with a chair, into which he collapses. He carries on shouting abuse at Karen.

Karen remains calm. She faces Robert and, keeping out of arm's length, squats down in front of him. She says nothing about the incident, but allows Robert to shout at her a little more. Gradually he begins to lower his voice, and rather than shouting at Karen he is beginning to talk, albeit loudly. She nods her head several times at what he is saying and when he pauses for a moment she says that he looks as if he is suffering inside, but under the circumstances he is handling the situation very well. Robert says of course he is suffering, and what would she know about it anyway. He is still angry, but he is no longer shouting. Karen continues to let him talk without interrupting him. After a couple of minutes she suggests to him that they have a cup of coffee and discuss ways that they can tackle his feelings without having more medication. He agrees, but says he still wants to see the doctor. Karen says that she realizes this and will make enquires as to when this can be arranged.

The key features of PE intervention are all present here, using the AIRS principles. Firstly, the nurse assessed the client's mental state, his stress factors and the risk factors involved. As a consequence of gaining that information she chose the moment to intervene actively, using the method which was most appropriate, resolved the actual emergency, and having reduced all the risk factors down to a more tolerable level she used supportive measures to maintain the link she had established. A frightening, and potentially dangerous situation for the nurse to be in, but one which is all too familiar. Yet the nurse dealt with it in a calm and rational way, enabling her to get on with the process of caring, and the client with the process of getting himself sorted out without losing his dignity.

This description of Karen's work outlines her direct interventions, but these in turn were supported by indirect interventions, and these need to be discussed in more detail before progressing any further.

Environmental considerations – indirect intervention

In the example Robert made to grab Karen, but she was able to step out of the way. The chair that Robert sat in, the space around which enabled Karen to stay where she wanted to be, and the vicinity of exit doors and other members of staff were not mentioned, but all of these were considerations which Karen had to deal with in making her decisions. Good environmental management within the emergency situation can only be achieved if the nurse remains alert and vigilant. It may require a conscious effort to view yourself within the space occupied by you and the client, and to consider all the possibilities that may ensue. Add to these the places and roles of those others who may be involved, other clients' relatives, family members and friends, visitors, other professionals as well as nurses, even workmen re-decorating the clinical area. Any one of them might be a significant player in the incident and will therefore need to be placed into this environmental framework that has to be used as the nurse's mental point of reference.

There are certain aspects of the nurse's response to an emergency which will be governed by environmental factors. There is no way that any nurse can legislate all the time for a client suddenly deciding to cut his wrists, or throwing himself out of a window, but certainly good planning prior to such an event would restrict the client to fewer opportunities for carrying out such actions. However, once they have occurred, or are being threatened which is often more likely to be the case, then the nurse has to make use of whatever environmental advantages exist. Manipulating an individual, who is threatening to take their own life, to move away from a stairwell, without alerting them either to its danger, or the intention of the nurse, is an extremely skilled activity. However, it is one which will not take place if the nurse fails to take account of his/her surroundings, and to use those surroundings to enhance direct interventions.

Using the environment, whether it be within an institutional, community or home setting, to reinforce the nurse's actions should be seen as dynamic process, arguably one of indirect intervention. It bears a resemblance to the place that non-verbal behaviour has when used as a method of reinforcing verbal behaviour. Either one used on their own may be quite effective, but when used together are far more potent and forceful.

AIRS principles – direct intervention

The concepts of Assessment, Intervention, Resolution and Support (AIRS) represent the four key elements to successfully tackling a psychiatric emergency. What we shall do in this section is look closely at each element, consider them in relation to a series of examples, and then integrate them to evaluate how they function within the immediate confines of the high-stress, high-risk environment of the PE.

Assessment

You may well ask the question, 'If I walk into a room and find a client sitting on his bed cutting himself repeatedly with a knife, what time have I got to carry out an assessment?' This seems a perfectly legitimate question to ask, but is it? Such a question assumes that the process of assessment begins only on finding the client when he is in the process of mutilating himself. It ignores the fact that the nurse will have initiated assessment procedures from the moment contact was made with the client as an inherent part of his nursing process, which in itself would have been continuously monitored, assessed and re-evaluated. It also assumes that the process of assessment is a long-winded and cumbersome exercise which takes up a lot of time and resources. It overlooks the fact that most assessments are made on a brief observation basis, and that assessment itself is often a re-appraisal of a situation, rather than an initiating procedure. Perhaps most seriously of all, however, it assumes that an assessment in such a situation is not necessary, thus denying nursing intervention any objective or rationale, and the client, recourse to the care quality necessary for the positive resolution of this emergency (Whittington and Wykes 1994).

Kupchik (1985) identifies seven key clinical areas for assessment within what he refers to as a 'disturbed behaviour situation'. These include an analysis of the precipitating crisis, the client's strengths and abilities and the working relationship between client and nurse. Both Getz (1980) and Hodgkinson (1980) felt it was more important to train carefully, rather than have clearly defined assessment tools, while Davis (1991) states, in his review of the literature on the subject of violence, that confusion exists about just what causes, and what defuses, such events. Very often the situations being discussed by these and other authors are not those requiring immediate emergency intervention, but more the crisis intervention events described in Chapter 1. Hence the seven areas described by Kupchik would be too cumbersome for a nurse to use if a client began kicking and scratching him for no apparent reason.

What does the literature on this subject tell us then? It shows the importance of nurses making up their own minds about what to look for when they find themselves in difficult or demanding situations. The rationale for this is quite simple. If you have had to work something out for yourself then you are far more likely to remember it than if someone simply gives it to you and tells you to get on with it. Maybe that is true, but it is always helpful to consider some alternatives beforehand. The following would be a reasonable focus to begin with.

• What does the client want?
• Who is in danger?
• What has caused this behaviour?

And, if the person is already known to you,

• What has happened in previous situations like this?
• What did this mean to the client the last time it happened?

You would also need to assess what resources were available to you, both personal and professional, like whether you felt you could cope, and whether or not there were other members of staff close by who could assist you if you called out to them.

These are questions you would answer very quickly. The answers you provide may not necessarily be totally accurate, but then that is hardly surprising. We are talking about one to two seconds here, and a rough approximation is as close as you can hope for. The answers you give will provide you with the basis for the action you take. You may only have a few seconds to get yourself out of a client's firm grip, or to stop someone from harming themselves.

You may feel that the questions posed above are helpful, but you might like to explore some alternatives. If this is the case ask yourself the question, 'If I were suddenly to be grabbed from behind by someone I did not know, and in a place where I could not get help, what would I need to know about my assailant to be able to get away?' Once you had answered that question, then you would need to ask a second one, only this time about being grabbed from behind by a client whom you knew, and in a clinical environment which had potential for your assistance. Compare the two sets of answers. It is likely that you would be less frightened by the second situation than by the first, and just as likely that your responses to the second would be both more specific and client-oriented. Moreover, the answers to the second question are likely to be tempered by those you answered to the first. For example, if you said in the first situation that you would need to know how big the person was, what his intention was and if he meant to hurt you, might you answer the same to the second situation? Or would you ask, is he capable of hurting you, what has caused him to do this to you, and how can you protect yourself from getting hurt?

While real threats to personal safety definitely exist within a healthcare environment, the uncertainty one associates with an unprovoked attack in the street tends to be absent when it is transferred to a ward, or emergency room. This makes it no less violent, or frightening, but the assessment questions to be asked will be shaped by this fact. In the street you may never be able to answer the questions that run through your head; in the ward you have to.

There may be situations where you have slightly more time to establish what is happening. For example:

> For the last 20 minutes June has been sitting talking to Alan about his feelings towards himself. He is convinced that he is evil and has been responsible for much of the bad things that he has seen on the television news. He has been trying to tell June that as far as he is concerned if he had never lived then life would be much better for a great many people. Logically, if he stays alive then others will die because of him, therefore it would be much better if he were dead. June has known Alan for a few days and already knows that he has these self-destructive feelings. She has had the opportunity to discuss some of the issues with the rest of her team and between them they had decided that there was a possibility that Alan might become violent towards himself. They had also ascertained that when he was calm and relaxed he seemed less prone to talk of self-harm.

As June listened she realized that despite her calm and controlled responses towards him, Alan was making himself agitated and it seemed as if he were challenging himself to act out a violent event. June excused herself for a few moments, explaining that she had to ask someone something. She attracted the attention of another member of the team, quickly explained what was happening and asked her colleague to take over from her. This he did. He also changed the topic of conversation reasonably quickly, and suggested that he and Alan should move to a more comfortable part of the ward.

Alan relaxed as he moved about and became interested in the new topic of conversation. He was still troubled by his own thoughts but the change in staff member appeared to have interrupted his train of thought and provided him with the opportunity to make peace with himself for a little while.

June knew from her knowledge of Alan that he was moving into a potential emergency situation. She felt it was easier to help him come to terms with himself before he lost control of his actions. The team had already decided on a plan of action for such an event and the game plan was that if the member of staff involved with Alan felt that they would be unable to stop the chain of events building up some sort of disruption, then while they still had the chance to do so, they were to change places with a colleague. The role of this nurse would be to alter the whole pattern of both the direct and indirect intervention being offered, while still being supported by the original nurse, albeit in a passive observational role.

In effect June used all the items of assessment listed above, but then she had more time than would normally be the case, and she was looking to avert an emergency rather than deal with one. In most situations of emergency the most that the nurse can hope to do is answer the first three questions. What does the client want? Who is in danger? and What has caused this behaviour?

Intervention

The information assessed by the nurse in those few seconds at the beginning of an emergency situation will form the basis of what is done to sort it out. However, there are two stages to this nursing action phase. The first of these is that of intervention, the second is resolution.

Intervention in some psychiatric settings is very difficult to define, because the rather seamless line between various nursing actions makes it difficult to establish when assessment has become planning, or intervention has become evaluation. Certainly the majority of nursing contact with clients has an interventionist quality about it no matter what the clinical intention. In a PE situation this is almost always the case. Yet, it is easier to identify the intervention required for the emergency, than it is for day-to-day clinical actions.

In a sense intervention is a form of mediation. The nurse has to mediate between the client's needs and the reality of what is available; mediate between the client's thoughts and beliefs about him/herself and the thoughts that may be haunting them, and mediate between danger and safety. Perhaps only during an emergency situation are all three of these forms of mediation required at the same time, and, if for no other reason, this makes the intervention all the more critical.

Whatever the nurse chooses to do it has to be carried out reasonably quickly; has to be concise and unambiguous, and it must be seen to be carried out in a confident and calm fashion. The specific intervention for each event will be determined by the nature of the event itself. For example, the nurse will respond differently if s/he is at the centre of an incident and therefore directly involved, than if it is one which is observed from a distance, rendering the nurse indirectly involved. What follows here is an outline of key points that may, when used either individually, or as part of a pattern, form the basis of an effective interventionist strategy. More specific applications are discussed in the practice Chapters 5–11.

The 'do's' of a psychiatric emergency

In any PE the nurse must do the following.

- Protect yourself from harm or danger. This may mean locking yourself in a cupboard and shouting for help, but at least you are safe.
- Always do something about the incident. You cannot observe it as if you are not involved – you are!
- Use whichever conflict resolution strategy you think is most suitable. Make the decision to use and do it. Do not question whether it was the right decision half way through the event. If it is obviously wrong, you will know because it will have no effect. The likelihood of making matters worse is a possibility, but they are already bad, so keep trying. Remember, there is no one right approach.

- Try and stay at arm's length from a potentially violent or aggressive client. Trying to grapple with a person, or risking the possibility of being hit or kicked just for the sake of seeming unafraid is a needless activity.
- Tell other staff where you are, and if necessary organize a support system or backup facility.
- Approach the client slowly, and try to keep your voice as calm as possible. Sometimes this can be achieved by breathing out before speaking, and selecting small sentences to speak. Because you do not have lungs full of air, your speech becomes easier to control. Some people find it easier to control their voice if they count to ten slowly before they speak, but you may not have the time to do this.
- Speak slowly and deliberately. If possible lower your voice so that the client has to listen more carefully to hear what you are saying. Try to speak in as deep voice as possible.
- Adopt a 'matter of fact' tone to your voice. Sometimes this has the effect of diffusing the client's emotional tension.
- Try to convey a sense of caring. This may be achieved through your physical presence and non-verbal behaviours, such as your posture, maintenance of appropriate eye contact and regular nodding of your head in response to what the client is saying, and by the use of empathetic phrases which indicate to the client that you really are paying attention to the pain they may be suffering. An example of such a statement would be, 'I can see that this is a difficult time for you, but you are doing extremely well under the circumstances.'
- Try to be unshockable. If you show that something upsets you or embarrasses you, the client may well concentrate on using it to abuse you.
- Try to distract the client if you feel that s/he will benefit from a time-out from the cause of the emergency.
- Conversely, you may decide to focus on the issues that have brought about the incident, allowing the client the opportunity to get it out of their system rather than bottling it all up inside.
- Allow the client to vent their feelings as much as you can, supporting them using effective non-verbal behaviour. If this means letting them shout and gesticulate, this is OK but you may need to consider other clients' feelings. Asking the client having the emergency to move to a place where s/he will

cause less concern to others may be an ideal solution, but the suggestion may well provoke further abuse, so be careful how you ask. It may be easier to ask the other clients to move.

- Summon the support of others if you feel that you cannot cope. There is no disgrace involved in admitting your limitations; in fact it is a recognition that you are in control of your actions.
- Try to separate clients who are fighting each other.
- If you have to use restraint ensure that there are the required number of staff to make the procedure safe for both the client and the staff. Name badges, neck ties rings and jewellery should be removed before carrying out such action. Restraint should be a last resort, but if carried out correctly and used as a mediation method, rather than a punitive response to aggression, it may still be an effective measure.
- If you are grabbed, or your clothing is held, move towards the client rather than trying to resist. If the attack is particularly threatening to you, try and get down on to the floor where it will be more difficult for your assailant to hold on to you.
- Try to fend off a really serious attacker by placing or holding something between you and the client. This may be an upturned chair, a table or some other item of furniture, but remember, it may be better to hold light or fragile objects in front of you, rather than leave them on the floor and have the client kick them at you. Don't worry about what you think you look like holding a chair out in front of you. If you are in this sort of a situation your appearance is the least of your worries.
- Always treat the client with respect and dignity, no matter what form of intervention you have to use.

The 'don'ts' of a psychiatric emergency

Inevitably there are certain things which nurses should not do in a PE situation, irrespective of the nature of the event, or the client involved. The following is a group of such actions, but nurses may find on some occasions that they have to do some of these because they simply have no other options. With one or two exceptions this may be acceptable but in the case of the first example this would never be tolerated.

- Never retaliate against a client, and certainly never strike a client no matter what the provocation.
- Do not try to manhandle a client, and if possible do not touch him/her at all.
- Do not belittle a client's outburst, or be seen to be laughing at him/her in any way. While this may seem an unusual tactic, sometimes when confronted by danger some people overcome their feelings by laughing.
- Do not let a client stand between you and your means of exiting a room or building. If the situation becomes difficult for you and you have lost the option to get out and get help, you are putting yourself in even more danger.
- Do not say things which could be taken the wrong way. Think about what you are going to say before saying it. You may only have the opportunity to make one statement to avert an emergency, so it needs to be a good one.
- Do not expect the client to be able to respond to what you ask him/her to do. They may be far too tense and agitated even to appreciate the words you are saying so do not be surprised if they appear not to hear you, or carry on doing what they are doing. It is not defiance, it is an inability to use cognitive reasoning. Modify your requests so that they can be more fully understood.
- Do not respond to personal abuse. It is all too easy to get angry with someone who is unpleasant towards you, but it will depreciate your clinical credibility with the client, and reduce your own confidence because you have lost control. Some experienced practitioners may be seen to argue with certain clients, but do not misinterpret this as a loss of control. It is a calculated strategy based on previous experience and professional confidence. It is not a strategy that should be adopted by the junior or less experienced nurse.
- Do not leave a client who is experiencing a PE on their own. In the event that the client requests such an action, and it is obvious that such a time-out might help them, the level of observation, support and accessibility of the client all need to be taken into consideration. In effect you do not leave the client alone, you reduce the level of contact to one which is more tolerable for the client.

- Do not act before you have to, or do more than is necessary to resolve the situation. In the long term 'over-intervening' can be as ineffective as 'under-intervening'.

While the physical purpose of these intervention principles is to save life or prevent injury the psychosocial purpose is threefold:

1. to have a direct impact on the client's ability to deal with their emotional state;
2. to give the client, as well as the nurse, the opportunity to get something positive out of this interaction;
3. to restore the client's confidence in him/herself.

Any action taken in an emergency situation must be measured against these outcomes. If the motive for strategy selection does not meet these requirements then it must be rethought during an evaluative or debriefing session.

Resolution

The second stage of the intervention section is that of resolution. It implies that the intervention has had a positive effect and that outcomes have been met. Most important of all it indicates that the client has been able to meet their immediate needs, and while there may still exist some element of danger, the situation has become less critical. Although this is still considered part of the PE this post-emergency stage requires a different set of skills to those already used. The nurse may not necessarily have a great deal of time to establish the nature of the resolution, but certain factors will indicate that it has taken place.

For a start the client's general demeanour will have altered, and no matter what the PE was they will be calmer and more relaxed. Their breathing will be more controlled, and where they have been shouting the tone of the voice begins to change, though it may not return to conversational levels for quite some time. At this point the nurse has to provide confirmation messages, that it is safe for the client to feel better, or acceptable to feel relieved. The client may still feel great anger or resentment so the nurse must at all costs avoid sounding patronizing. Positive reassurance, and connectiveness are required here, while at the same time carrying out a re-assessment of the client's mental state (Lowe 1992).

Points to consider at this stage include the following.

- What are the client's behaviour and mental state prior to the PE?
- What are the changes that have taken place since the height of the PE?
- What is the apparent intent of the client at this stage?
- What are his/her body mechanics, such as breathing, movement, eye contact etc.?
- How have your confirmation messages been received?
- What is his/her speech content?
- Are intellectual functions returning to their pre-PE levels?
- What level of judgement is being expressed?
- What is the potential for destructive behaviour?
- What level of psychological disturbance exists?
- Do not leave the client on his/her own.
- Do not assume that the client is all right now.
- Have the intervention outcomes been met? These must be measured in some way.
- Arrange for another team member to take over from you if you think it would be appropriate.

The key points relate to meeting the client's needs, and achieving the intervention outcomes. Of course, not all PEs will require such a large amount of analysis. For example:

Michael is being visited by his girl friend. He wants her to stay in the hospital because he is lonely. She cannot do this and refuses. He becomes very angry, accuses her of not loving him and abandoning him in the hospital. He shouts that she is being unfaithful to him and starts to call her insulting names. Jack, his primary nurse, has been watching all this and decides that it is time to intervene. He asks Michael, in a reasonably matter-of-fact way, who has been making all the noise. Michael repeats some of what he has been saying. Jack asks the girlfriend to wait there for a little while and says to Michael that if he feels that way then he and Jack ought to go and do something else. Ten minutes later, halfway through making a cup of coffee, Michael, who has not mentioned the incident, says that he really misses his girlfriend, and was wrong to shout at her. Jack asks him what he is going to do about it, and Michael walks back to his girlfriend full of apologies.

Jack simply monitored Michael's voice level, and non-verbal behaviour. He knew that this had happened before and he also guessed that if it was handled without confrontation it could be resolved by Michael himself. Jack knew that the matter had been resolved because he asked for confirmation from Michael.

Support – for the client

Of course, once he had returned to his girlfriend Michael was still being carefully observed by Jack who, after a time, went over to the couple and asked them how they were getting on together. He listened to what they had to say and spent some time with them acting as a sort of arbitrator till they were happy with their decisions. In effect, Jack was giving Michael the support he needed to be able to think more clearly and reach a more satisfactory arrangement with his girlfriend.

Support is essentially a post-emergency stage. It gives the nurse the opportunity to measure the effects of intervention, but it also allows the client time to reflect on the incident and regain their composure. It is crucial that they have time in which to recapture some of their self-respect. It is not unusual for clients to become tearful or remorseful after experiencing a PE, and for obvious reasons. Having lost control of their emotional state, or found themselves overwhelmed by feelings of anger and frustration, many clients encounter feelings of loss, while others feel that they have let themselves down and that others will be critical of them.

The nurse has to be prepared to spend time with the client in an attempt to help them regain personal confidence or, in the absence of this, at least to enable them to come to terms with what has happened. The nurse must nurture the positive devel-opments that have arisen as a consequence of the PE both by reassuring the client of their safety and discussing the event in a non-judgemental fashion. Manglass (1986) talks of providing emotional support, and certainly this would appear to be the main purpose of this stage of AIRS.

The method of support will vary from client to client, and there will be those who need to be left to sort things out for themselves. Support in this case is knowing when to be involved and when to leave alone. However, no matter what form of support is necessary the client must spend some time with the nurse, even if it serves only as a period of reconciliation (Emrich 1989).

Support – for the nurse

It is certainly not uncommon to find nurses, and other care professionals, who have had to deal with a PE experiencing a personal reaction afterwards. The response will vary according to the situation, the nurse's involvement and his/her appreciation of what took place. It could include feelings of anger or frustration, embarrassment or impatience. They could be frightened, belligerent, nauseated, find it difficult to concentrate, but most will have an overwhelming desire to talk about the event (Hartsough and Mayers 1985).

Many will feel that they could have done better during the incident, while others will see themselves as failing to detect the change in a client's behaviour that would have indicated a PE was imminent. Probably worse still are those who blame themselves for the whole event. In just about every case their fears about their performance may be totally unfounded, yet one of the main reasons for providing support facilities for these nurses is not to help them build confidence, but to give them the opportunity to vent their feelings and relieve their emotional tension.

Those responsible for this support, be they clinical supervisors, mentors or peers, must encourage the nurse not only to recount the events of the PE but also to be honest about their feeling concerning the incident. The rebuilding of personal confidence cannot take place until the conflicts concerning this event have been met head on and tackled to the nurse's satisfaction. A nurse who truly has been responsible for a PE occurring has to be given the time out to explore what went wrong, but that restructuring process can only happen once the incident itself has been confronted and accepted.

Nurses must feel safe to talk about their experiences, safe from ridicule and safe from harsh judgement, especially from those who were not present during the incident (Thompson

1992). See Chapter 12 for a more detailed discussion on staff support.

The final part of the support stage is an evaluation of the event, usually by peers, supervisors or clinical teams, to see if anything can be learnt from how the event was dealt with (Dang 1990). This is not an exercise in finding blame. On the contrary, it may well be that the team wish to congratulate nurses on their performance, and to show their support for the actions that were taken. However, it is important that those carrying out the review, usually the peers of those involved, need to recognize that there is a vast difference between the wisdom of hindsight, as practised in the calm light of a new day, and the heat and desperation experienced at the flashpoint of a life and death event. Tolerance and professional reality must be combined to produce realistic guidelines for future intervention.

Conclusion

The PE is something that can only be partially prepared for. In most cases there is no single correct way of dealing with it, and most nurses who feel that they might have been able to prevent it had they done something else are usually wrong. Others express feelings of uncertainty about their ability to identify behaviours that lead to a PE. Similarly, nurses who become involved in PE events sometimes feel that they will make matters worse and lose the confidence to do anything at all. The fact is that things cannot get much worse than they already are, so the nurse might as well do something! PEs are often unstoppable, or would require super human resources and insight to be able to predict and manage. Nurses are human and must accept the limitations this imposes

The introduction of an AIRS-based strategy is one way of providing a baseline for practice. It offers a series of elements which piece together to form a systematized approach to PE intervention and resolution. It has to be an approach adopted by all the members of the clinical team if it is to be effective, and the corporate approach has in turn to be supported by effective evaluative and after-care services. Nurses need to support each other and help each other through difficult-to-manage situations. If a nurse chooses a method of intervention different their colleagues, this does not make them wrong, simply different.

References

Dang, S. (1990). When the patient is out of control. *RN*, 53(10):57–8.

Davis, S. (1991). Violence by psychiatric patients: a review. *Hospital and Community Psychiatry*, 42(6):585–90.

Emrich, K. (1989). Helping or hurting? Interacting in the psychiatric milieu. *Journal of Psychosocial Nursing and Mental Health Services*, 27(12).

Gertz, B. (1980). Training for prevention of assaultive behaviour in a psychiatric setting. *Hospital and Community Psychiatry*, 31:628–30.

Hartsough, D. M. and Mayers, D. G. (1985). *Disaster Work and Mental Health: Prevention and Control of Stress among Workers*. Rockville, MD, National Institute of Mental Health, Washington.

Hodgkinson, P. (1980). Psychological approaches to violence. *Nursing Times*, 76(32):1399–1401.

Kupchik, D. (1985). Prevention and management of disturbed behaviour: *Psychiatric Nursing*, Oct./Nov./Dec., 85: 9–11.

Lowe, T. (1992). Characteristics of effective nursing interventions in the management of challenging behaviour. *Journal of Advanced Nursing*, 17: 1226–32.

Manglass, L. (1986). Psychiatric interventions you can use in a crisis. *RN*, 49(11):38–9.

Norris, M. K. and Kennedy, C. W. (1992). The view from within: how patients perceive the seclusion process. *Journal of Psychosocial Nursing and Mental Health Services*, 30(3):7–13.

Thompson, J. (1992). Stress theory and therapeutic practice. *3rd International Society for the Investigation of Stress Conference*. London University College and Middlesex Hospital School of Medicine, Middlesex Hospital, London.

Weaver, S. M., Brooke, A. K. and Kat, B. J. B. (1978). Some patterns of disturbed behaviour in a closed ward environment. *Journal of Advanced Nursing*, 3:251–63.

Whittington, R. and Wykes, T. (1994). An observational study of associations between nurse behaviour and violence in psychiatric hospitals. *Journal of Psychiatric and Mental Health Nursing*, 1(2):85–92.

Suggested reading

Connolly, M. J. (1992). Issues and developments in psychiatric nursing: history. Chapter 2 in Brooking, J. I., Ritter, S. A. H. and Thomas, B. L. (eds), *A Textbook of Psychiatric and Mental Health Nursing*, Churchill Livingstone, Edinburgh. (Gives a good description of how mental health nursing has developed and why it should be that some early nurses behaved the way that they did.)

Dreyfus, J. K. (1987). Nursing assessment of the ED patient with psychiatric symptoms: a quick reference. *Journal of Emergency Nursing*, 13(5):278–82. (Essentially for nurses working in an acute general area, but the assessment process is an approach which might be useful in some PE situations.)

Stevenson, S. (1991). Heading off violence with verbal de-escalation. *Journal of Psychosocial Nursing and Mental Health Services*, 29(9):6–10, 36–7. (Uses case studies to explores the interaction between verbal and non-verbal strategies in potential PE situations.)

5

Emergencies associated with self-harm

Introduction

You do not have to have a psychiatric problem to generate a psychiatric emergency. We all have the capacity to harm ourselves, either intentionally or unintentionally, yet this does not necessarily mean that we are confronted by enormous emotional problems, nor does it mean that we wish to take our own lives. While it is true that poor mental health is likely to increase the potential for a PE, for those who undertake self-harm there may be other factors at play.

Self-harm is essentially some form of self-damaging behaviour which can be as serious as killing oneself, or less seriously, gestures designed to draw attention to oneself (Adam 1985). The term self-harm is not always used to describe the behaviours of such events. Self-injurious behaviour (SIB) as outlined by Carr (1977) can range from eating soil, to swallowing rat poison, to rubbing the face with rough cloth till it becomes red and swollen, to cutting wrists, or biting your nails till they bleed, to biting open old wounds and eventually bleeding to death. Self-destructive behaviour is a term that Adams (1985) uses to describe suicide, or attempted suicide. Stengel (1964) explored the differences between suicide and parasuicide, i.e. those who killed themselves, or attempted to, and those who mimic such actions but do not intend to kill themselves. Self-mutilation (Podvoll 1969), and minor self-injury (Ballinger 1971) outline more specific events. Then there are a whole range of sub-sections of self-harm which describe in more detail the nature of the behaviour, i.e. intentional self-harm, unintentional self harm, overdosing or self-poisoning, self-ligation, attention seeking behaviour, body abuse, threats to body abuse, scarification, self-abusive behaviour and post-injury crisis. The list is long, and the behaviours involved are often distressing, both for the observer and for those who undertake them.

The term self-harm is used here as a generic term to describe the process by which individuals intentionally either cause themselves physical damage or put themselves at risk of being harmed in some way.

Self-harm and mental health

Is it possible to reconcile the concept of self-harm with that of mental health? For those who have never experienced the depth of sadness or the intense distortion of reality that may be associated with clinical depression, the answer is probably no. Yet, most people only view self-harm from their own perception of how life should be ordered. 'You were given a body and this body is yours, but you have to look after it. If it goes wrong help will be provided to put it right, but if you damage it in some way and it goes wrong because of your actions then you will receive less help, because it is your fault. The body has to work properly at all costs.' A social psychologist might argue that such a shared belief would be important in maintaining individuals within a complex social setting (Abraham and Shanley 1992). Yet it also has the effect of making people think that because they would do nothing intentional to harm their own bodies, then it is in some way wrong if other people do it to themselves. Most religions see suicide as wrong, and in some countries of the world it is still illegal to kill yourself. Does it follow that if the majority of people say it is wrong to take your own life, and you go ahead and do it, or make a serious attempt at it, then you have done something wrong? More significantly, does it mean that there is something wrong with you?

To answer this question is important on two counts. Firstly, because by answering it we should develop a better understanding of why we behave the way we do towards people who behave differently to ourselves, and secondly, because by having that better knowledge we may then be able to determine a more effective way of intervening in PE situations generated by clients who are self-harming.

It is almost impossible to imagine the sense of desperation that many potential suicides experience, while others feel relieved at the sense of certainty the decision to end it all brings. However, what we can do is focus on the interactive circumstances that may occur. For example, if you saw no future in your life, no meaning or purpose for it, felt that all the alternatives were closed to you or you felt so responsible for something terrible that had happened and you just could not contend with the guilt it left, what would you do about it? You might seek help from a healthcare professional, yes, but to do so would require you to perceive your feelings as being related to health. Few people see guilt, sadness or intense emotional distress as being a health problem, especially when it is they who are experiencing it. You might see a priest, but these days formal religion plays less part in many people's lives and you might not think it appropriate to seek help from such an institution. Friends and relatives do not help. Oh, they try, looking concerned and embarrassed when you talk to them, but they have as much difficulty coping with your expression of your feelings as you do experiencing them. Others are insensitive towards you, seeing you as weak and telling you that you would be all right if only you would take a holiday. They do not realize that you would take the pain and guilt on the package tour with you, and besides, you do not necessarily want to feel better. What you want is answers, and in particular the answer to the question, what do I do with my thoughts and feelings?

Under such circumstances, where no-one appears to be able to offer an alternative, where no-one even seems to have an understanding of your various dilemmas, is it really strange that you should consider the possibility of taking your own life. Once the thought has entered your head, you would find it difficult to get rid of it. For many the deliberate planning that goes into their suicide is an acceptance of their fate, while for others it is a spontaneous response to the desire for peace, or even punishment. Then, either out of sheer frustration at your own inability, or the search for the final solution, you kill yourself. Under these circumstances does suicide, or its attempt, sound so irrational? Even if it does, does it sound more understandable? Being able to make sense of what the client is doing provides you with a better opportunity for informed decisions to intervene on their behalf.

For most nurses the concept of intentional self-harm is associated with people experiencing a mental health problem. Within medical or surgical environments those problems may well have been brought about by their physical condition, or their inability to cope with the condition. Relationships with fellow patients, staff and visitors may all help to provoke a sense of desperation and loneliness that sees them hurting themselves in some way. If the nurse sees this behaviour in a negative way and chooses not to explore the reasons for it then the interventions used to intervene at the time of a PE will be both ineffective and professionally unsatisfactory.

So far we have only considered the most obvious of self-harm acts, that of suicide, but there are any number of less obvious ones that people may use as a release from the pressure they feel. True, a great many of them either occur in the person's home rather than in a hospital setting, and when they do occur in hospitals it usually psychiatric ones, but that does not necessarily mean that all individuals who choose to hurt themselves in some way have mental health problems. What it means is that most of them inflict wounds or injuries that are not serious enough to warrant medical attention. A great many people get angry and become violent towards 'things' rather than people, with the result that the 'things', being considerably harder than they are, cause minor injury. Transitory psychological distress is something from which all of us suffer from one time or another, but it has little or no long-term effect. The release of pent-up emotional energy at such times is common and, despite the possible damage it causes to heads and hands, often necessary.

Self-harm and the psychiatric emergency

When the self-harm behaviour is such that it threatens life, or puts the individual at risk, or there are accompanying mental health problems, then it may well constitute a psychiatric emergency. Unlike other PEs, however, many of the self-harm situations are more insidious. They do not occur as a single flashpoint, but more as a series of events which lead up to the incident. The implication of this for nurses is that it provides the opportunity to intervene at several stages in the procedure. The skill is knowing not only what to say and do, but when to do it.

The style of intervention will also differ from the more abrupt form of PE. For example, talking in a quiet, almost whispered voice to someone contemplating suicide, may well be effective, but talking to someone who is self-mutilating their arm with a razor blade will probably have little or no effect at all. The potential suicide may be seeking your help and may wish to be talked out of hurting themselves, while the self-mutilator will stop only when s/he is ready to do so.

A PE involving self-harm may be life threatening in itself, but once the client has taken some serious action against him/herself it often becomes a medical emergency as well. However, some self-harm behaviours, while constituting a PE, do not necessarily generate so much risk for the client who indulges in them. Ferry (1992) identified a list of some 20 self-injurious behaviours (SIB) in his study of people with learning disabilities in Rampton Special Hospital, England. The list includes such things as air swallowing and self-cutting. Some of these behaviours, while obviously causing alarm, would not in themselves constitute an emergency. SIBs generating this level of concern would be those which directly affect the client's ability to maintain life support. They would include self-cutting, depending on the severity of the cut, burning or biting oneself, head-banging and self-poisoning.

Burrow (1992) also highlights another key issue concerning self-harm of this intensity. He argues that self-harm itself is expressed among healthcare professionals as being intentional, and as such the client is held responsible. This differs from other pathological behaviours, such as violence towards others, which are seen to be carried out by clients who are 'sick', and therefore cannot be held responsible for their actions. While Burrow offers no evidence of this, Hoff (1989) would appear to confirm this notion when he describes trying to understand people in crisis, rather than using judgemental interventions. Certainly Burrow's cautionary statement must be considered by nurses having to deal with self-harm PEs. If the nurse believes that clients hurt themselves intentionally and not as a consequence of intense emotional stress, that the act of self-poisoning is simply to draw attention to themselves, or that they are only cutting themselves because they enjoy pain, then what kind of intervention will be offered? The problem is that if the nurse has these beliefs then the act of self-harming becomes devalued. It is almost as if the nurse is saying that some behaviours are real and are committed by those who are mentally ill, while others are not real, no matter how serious, and are committed by those who are not mentally ill. The care offered to the two groups will undoubtedly be of differing quality, because the nurse will believe that for the first group she is doing something for people who cannot help themselves and are therefore genuine, while for the second group she will be helping people who could have helped themselves, are therefore not genuine, and are taking advantage of her.

It is obvious that such beliefs and attitudes must not interfere with a nurse's perception of her obligation to a self-harming client in a PE, but it is difficult to overcome such beliefs if they are present (van den Bent-Kelly 1992). In truth the nurse has to try to make sense of the client's behaviour from the client's point of view, rather than from the nurse's. This requires patience, skill and a real desire to understand what is happening. However, the end result is a better understanding of what is required, and better care delivery at the point of contact with the client. It is important that the nurse admits to such beliefs, because until such time as s/he does so then it will be impossible to achieve the results described above. The nurse will derive no satisfaction from working with the self-harming client, and that too will interfere with their performance. Unfortunately, all too often nurses are aware that others have these beliefs, know that they have a detrimental effect on care, yet by denying they also have them, convince themselves that they are doing the best they can (Pederson 1993). The longer this belief is reinforced, the more difficult it will become for the nurse to change, while all the time, the self-harming client is receiving what is essentially second-class intervention.

Self-harm and AIRS

The incidence of self-harm, especially suicide, is increasing within the UK, along with the rest of the developed world. This applies to both the older person (Courage *et al.* 1993, Etzersdorf and Fischer 1993), young people in the community (Hawton and Fagg 1992, Sonneborn and Vamstraelen 1992) and both genders (Brant and Osgood 1990, Evans and Lacey 1992, Nowers 1993). The implications of this for nurses is that while certain clinical specialities have always had to deal with more PEs than others, these days no speciality can be said to be without the potential for such events. Few nurses are given adequate training within their educational development to be able to handle PEs effectively, so it is necessary for them to equip themselves with a game plan, in this case the AIRS approach.

It would be impossible to explore all the ramifications of AIRS interventions for all the self-harm behaviours, so I have elected to explore three separate incidents. In themselves they will offer a variety of personal approaches, and will give some indication of the differences that exist within the self-harm PE. However, they do not represent in any way everything that may be done in such circumstances, but act as an example of what is possible.

Clients who put themselves at risk

While a few people actively seek danger for recreational purposes, most of us spend the majority of our lives actively avoiding it. Yet for some there comes a time when life appears so terrible that they not only seek danger, but set out to hurt themselves, or even take their own lives. The following examples explore PEs for three people who fall into this group. They have been chosen because they give the opportunity to consider the use of AIRS in vastly different self-harm scenarios, and not because they are the most common or most serious. The reader is reminded that the interventions described are not exclusive to such situations.

Patricia – an elderly lady putting herself at risk

Patricia has recently been admitted to an assessment unit because her behaviour has caused concern. She is 72 and has been a widow for six years. She has been living with her daughter for the last two years and for most of that time everything seems to have been all right. Over the last few months she has become increasingly forgetful and her daughter has come home from work to find her mother crying on several occasions. Patricia appeard to be getting distressed for no apparent reason and frustrated when she is unable to express her feelings. It is obvious that she is becoming isolated from her friends and relatives and is unhappy with her personal circumstances.

What has worried the daughter is that Patrica has developed a habit of doing things which seem out of character and, in some instances, quite dangerous. On one cold day she was found gardening wearing only flimsy summer clothing, and on another occasion she failed to return from a stroll and was discovered wandering aimlessly and crying in a nearby park. Over the past couple of weeks she has knocked and bruised herself and had to be taken to the local A&E department, because she fell heavily while out shopping. She seems to be aware of the distress she is causing her daughter but tells her not to be concerned because 'It will be all right soon.'

The GP is unable to determine just how much of Patricia's behaviour she is controlling herself, and the CPN to whom she was referred felt that there was an element of intent in some of the self-harm actions. Since being admitted she has appeared reasonably cheerful, and has willingly participated in her assessment. However, the nurses report that on more than one occasion she seems to be distracted and becomes preoccupied with certain courses of action.

This morning her primary nurse has detected a change in Patricia's mood. She is unhappy and talking of leaving the Unit. The nurse discusses this in depth with her, but Patricia becomes more determined to leave. She eventually gets up and walks away. The nurse decides to leave her alone for a while, feeling that perhaps their conversation has made things worse. The nurses discuss Patricia's current presentation, and in particular her judgement and mental state. They agree that her emotional distress is heavily influencing her decision to leave and decide to intervene in this area, rather than tackle the leaving issue. However, before they have time to put this strategy into action, a visitor reports that Patricia has just pushed past her at the Unit entrance and is headed for the main road.

When the nurse reaches her she finds Patrica standing at a stop for a bus which goes in the wrong direction. She is distressed and looking about her in an agitated fashion. The nurse realizes that she cannot simply ask Patricia to come back with her, and the situation is complicated by the other people waiting for the bus who are wary of the whole situation.

Patricia is only wearing a nightdress, and when she sees the nurse shouts at her that if she comes any closer she will jump into the path of the oncoming bus.

The PE confronting the nurse is that Patricia is placing herself at risk from jumping into the traffic, not the on-going problem of her desire to leave. In this situation the nurse has to remember that although the two issues are connected, her main concern is to stop Patricia from hurting herself, and to do so in such a way that Patricia does not lose any more dignity than she has. Simply grabbing hold of her and marching her back to the Unit is unacceptable, legally, professionally and morally. The nurse has to concentrate on the current situation and ignore other distractions, like her location and the possible protestations of the waiting passengers. The key to success in this situation stems from the conversation she has just had with her colleagues.

The nurse does not approach Patrica directly, but, moving slowly, and while talking as quietly as possible, gradually walks towards her. She ignores the well-meaning interruptions and advice from the other passengers and manages to get herself between Patricia and the bus-shelter exit which is next to the road. Having done so she is now able, if necessary, to stop Patricia from jumping into the road. Her first priority has been met, as Patricia is no longer able to hurt herself at this point. Her second priority is to get Patricia to calm herself enough to be able to talk more rationally about what she wants to do. The nurse remembers that their earlier conversation about leaving seemed to have made Patricia more determined to do so, and that her colleagues had decided to concentrate on a strategy designed to help Patricia feel more positive about herself. With this in mind she asks Patricia what she is doing. She asks her if she feels cold. She offers her the coat that she has brought with her, saying that she can borrow it for a while, telling Patricia that she looks very good in it.

She allows Patricia to talk for a while about what she is doing, not interrupting but nodding her head occasionally, and agreeing with her on several points. She compliments Patricia on several issues, especially her ability to cope with the way she is feeling. She suggests moving away from the queue, because she says she cannot not hear what Patricia is saying above the noise of the traffic. She accentuates this a little by leaning towards her, adopting a facial expression indicating concern, and speaks quietly so that Patricia also finds it difficult to hear her in return. Eventually they move back away from the road, with the nurse placing herself between Patricia and the kerb, which has the double effect of protecting her from the danger of the traffic and the prying eyes of the waiting queue. She initiates a conversation about something she has read in the newspaper that morning, and gradually Patricia becomes interested in what she is saying. Eventually the nurse suggests they both go and get a cup of tea as she is feeling very cold and she can see that Patricia is too. Slowly they return to the Unit arm in arm.

The assessment here was that of identifying the nature of the danger to Patricia, and those factors which seemed to have led up to the PE. The intervention was both direct and indirect, and though simplistic, had to contend with extraneous elements such as the location and bystanders. Ensuring that Patricia could not jump into the road was the major concern, but it was dealt with in a quiet and confident manner so that she was not frightened by the nurse. The topic of conversation could have been anything that the nurse felt relevant, just as long as it distracted thoughts of leaving the Unit, and was of a positive nature. The use of connectiveness, or shared experience, was invaluable in helping Patricia to feel that both she and the nurse were working together, and the empathetic responses of the nurse helped to reinforce this. The situation was resolved once this feeling of togetherness had been achieved. The final return to the Unit was achieved without any further loss of dignity, and walking arm in arm with Patricia enhanced the support the nurse offered (Ruthven 1987).

Of course, not all PEs occur in the public eye as this one did, but when they do the nurse has to be conscious of protecting the client both from their own actions and the potential interference, or even hostility, of onlookers. Such a balance is difficult to achieve, but can only be done so by putting the client's needs first.

Tony – who cuts himself

Some PEs are difficult to foresee, as with the previous example, while others may occur regularly as part of a client's pattern of response to stress or emotional tension. In the following example the PE described only involves two people, Mike, the primary nurse, and Tony a 23-year-old who has a long history of self-mutilation. The circumstances of the PE have been experienced several times before and while Mike is alone with Tony on this occasion, the collective skills of the whole clinical team have produced the AIRS approach that he adopts.

Mike knew that something was wrong even before he entered the room. Usually the radio would be on quite loud and the door would be open slightly allowing the occupant to see what was going on outside. This morning it was quiet and the door closed. Mike knocked several times before any reply came from within. As he walked in he was struck by the silence once again, but more so by the young man sitting cross-legged on the bed in front of him, his shirt sleeves rolled up and blood running down his forearms. Tony did not bother to look up but simply made another cutting stroke of his left arm. Mike counted a dozen other cuts as well as the countless scars from similar previous episodes.

'I came to see how you were,' he said, knowing that he would get no reply. He moved over to the chair by the side of the bed and sat down. He said no more and simply watched, and waited. Tony was breathing heavily and concentrating on the razor blade in his hand. No-one could work out how he managed to get razor blades so easily, but he always had one when he wanted to do this to himself. At first the nurses had blamed themselves for failing to detect them, but soon realized that he would eventually get something to cut himself with no matter what they did.

After a short pause, and before Tony cut himself again, Mike said, 'Now that I am here do you want to tell me what you are feeling inside?' Tony said that he did not, but he did say that he wanted to be left alone. He knew that Mike would not leave. Mike said in a matter-of-fact way that he could remember what Tony had said the last time this happened, that he had said he could not control himself and that it was the only way he could release the terrible pressure he felt inside of himself. Tony said that it was the same again. 'Have you any idea what brought it on this time?' Mike asked. Tony had not, but he was prepared to tell him just how bad he felt, and how miserable everything was. Mike told him that under the circumstances he felt Tony had done extremely well to go so long between this episode and the last one. Tony looked up and smiled at him without any humour.

They talked about what Tony was feeling, and Mike reminded Tony that they had agreed that if Tony felt this way again he would talk to Mike before the feelings got so bad that he felt the urge to cut himself. Tony said that he remembered, but just could not stop himself. All the time they were talking he held the razor in his hand, but he was no longer cutting himself, and Mike behaved as if there was no blade. After a little while longer Mike asked Tony if he wanted to give it to him, and Tony did so. He started to sob and for the next half an hour Mike sat with him, saying little, simply sitting by the bed.

Mike's response to this PE was to remain as calm as possible. He had to assess the extent to which Tony had already cut himself, and the depth of the mood he was in. In deciding upon the course of action he took he had to take something of a risk. By not responding to the situation as if it were an emergency, he was trying to show Tony that he was not critical of him. Yet such a non-judgemental approach could have backfired on him because, having entered into this type of contract with Tony, what would he do if Tony decided to carry on cutting himself while Mike sat there? On this occasion it did not happen, but this was because Mike stayed calm and trusted in the approach the team had carefully worked out beforehand. He had to take the risk that Tony might cut again, and if he had, then Mike would have had to let him do it. He could not maintain the trust that Tony had in him if he had done otherwise. When would he have stopped him had the behaviour continued? He probably would not have physically stopped him but if his pre-determined intervention had been ineffective he would have had to adapt it on the spot so that it did have the desired effect. The resolution of this PE occurred when Tony made eye contact with Mike, because he decided that he no longer wanted to cut himself, and Mike had been there for him till he made that decision. The non-intrusive support which Mike gave after the event was crucial to any further therapeutic developments between them (Burrow 1992).

Derek – making a suicidal attempt

Most nurses do not have to deal directly with the attempt a client makes in taking their own life. The nurses' work is often confined to restoring clients' physical states, as in the work of A&E or trauma ward staff, developing future coping initiatives with liaison psychiatric nurses, or, in the case of most psychiatric nurses, providing special supervision and support during clinical depression in an attempt to stop such events taking place.

However, clients do try to take their own lives, even when they are undergoing intensive in-patient therapy. In fact, they are most at risk when care staff have been successful in raising clients' moods out of the deep depression that brought them into care in the first place. Nurses need to be aware that as clients' volitional impulses increase so too do they regain the motivational strength to carry out the self-destructive actions upon which they have been ruminating while depressed. This is a critical time for the client, and one for which the nurses must plan. It is too easy, as the following example shows, for nurses to regard limited recovery as reason for reducing supervision, when it should really be a signal for greater vigilance.

What this example also shows is the contrast between the intervention style adopted in the case of Tony, where risk-taking was a calculated part of the approach, and taking time was fundamental to its success, and the necessity to move swiftly and directly in Derek's case because he will undoubtedly kill himself if not.

Derek had been in hospital for three months. During that time he has been seriously depressed, communicating hardly at all for days on end, isolating himself from everyone and experiencing terrible and frightening thoughts about himself and his relationships with the world at large. He is 49-years-old and despite the fact that he has a loving, caring family, a good job and an apparently satisfying lifestyle, he can see no reason to carry on living. Within the last couple of days he has become more animated and the nurses in his team have reported that he is talking more, eating better and his sleep pattern has improved. The general feeling is that he is at last beginning to get better. The nurses have spent so much time with him that they have managed to build up a profile of how he feels and some of the thoughts that he is experiencing. They know that he is experiencing suicidal thoughts and his improvement in mood has alerted them to the necessity of ensuring that he does not have the opportunity to do anything about them. They are also aware that now he has regained some of his lost momentum he is very much more at risk. Consequently they have altered their observational status to include constant supervision, to continue till such time as they are more confident of his intentions.

They have also developed a handover policy among themselves which ensures that they are aware of his current thoughts and feelings. They recognize that if he is determined to harm himself they will need to respond rapidly if they are to stop him.

Despite all their caution Derek suddenly makes a dash for the door. The ward is on the first floor of the building and outside the door is an open stairwell. If he reaches it before the nurse he could easily throw himself headlong over it. The nurse has kept himself within arm's reach of Derek, but the swiftness of his movement has caught him off guard. It is a race to see who get to the stairs first!

Obviously if the nurse reaches the stairs before Derek, talking quietly to him and maintaining a non-intrusive contract with him will serve little purpose. He has to stop him from jumping, any way that he can. The purpose of his AIRS strategy is to maintain life, at any cost. His assessment of the situation is instant, Derek is going to harm himself; his intervention must be equally as instant.

As he runs the nurse shouts for assistance, but he is the closest and all will depend on him. Derek is held up a little as he reaches the door, while the nurse is able to bolt through rapidly as Derek leaves it open behind him. This enables the nurse to catch Derek before the stairwell and he grabs him firmly from behind halting his progress as he does so. Before Derek can alter his position and struggle free the nurse moves round in front of him, blocking his path, and holds his arms firmly around Derek's waist, pinning his arms to his sides. As he does so, the nurse talks to Derek, telling him that he is here, that he can talk to him and asking him not to do what he has tried to do.

They are joined by two other nurses, but they do not crowd in on the scene, nor do they touch Derek or try to hold him. They stand waiting to provide assistance and back-up support should the first nurse require it. If he can think of nothing positive to say, or if he needs help in deciding the best course of action, they will prompt him, but they will not take over from him unless he specifically asks them to.

The nurse reminds Derek of the tremendous progress he has made, of how impressed he is with the way Derek is coping with his thoughts and feelings, and how important he is to others. Most importantly, he does not let go, nor does he loosen his grip. Derek is not struggling and the nurse's hold on him has the effect of reinforcing the fact that he does not want him to kill himself. The nurse is not even looking at Derek, he has tucked in so closely that he is almost cradling him in his arms. Derek's face cannot be seen by the nurse, therefore Derek can experience his own pain of failure, without the indignity of being viewed doing so. The nurse must stay like this until Derek decides to return to the ward. Only by staying still and allowing Derek to grieve for himself will any resolution take place.

Eventually the nurse feels the tension decrease in Derek's body and they negotiate a return to the ward. They spend a great deal of the next hour sitting in silence as the nurse gently begins to prompt Derek as to why he did it, providing important information that might help the team to predict a further attempt, and giving Derek the opportunity to continue his recovery.

Perhaps the intervention in this PE is obvious, but it is the way that it is carried through which is of most significance. The same caring sense has to be conveyed to the client as in any other therapeutic encounter, but the sheer speed of the initial surge can inhibit this. The nurse has to overcome his own fears for the client, and the remainder of the team have to resist the temptation of interfering in the proceedings. The desire to save the client from harm could become a barrier to effective long-term intervention. In this case the nurse responsible for the intervention made all the decisions concerning resolution and support, but in cases where the nurse runs out of ideas, or just does not feel capable of making the decisions, it is perfectly acceptable for them to hand over to someone who can. Had such a case arisen here then the second nurse would have resumed the same position as the first, both in providing physical as well as psychological support during the resolution stage, and afterwards in the support stage itself. The physical support is important here, because sometimes it is just impossible to convey the sense of caring that people have for each other through word alone (Reid and Long 1993).

Conclusion

In this chapter we have explored the nature of PE in relation to self-harm and some of its many variations. We have seen that in some cases the intervention required is controlled and subtle, distracting in nature and dependent upon discreet direct and indirect approaches, while in other situations the approach is far more abrupt, demanding split-second action to avert disaster. We have seen that in certain situations nurses have to take calculated risks, but that previous knowledge of client behaviours and an exploration of the effects certain interventions have upon them, are crucial to the faith nurses have in their own decisions at times of crisis.

The use of the AIRS approach has been the common factor for all the situations, with each nurse, or team of nurses, using the four components to build their strategies. It has also been used to give nurses an appreciation of their performance through the emergency, acting as guide to what point the emergency has reached, and helping the nurse work systematically through the challenge of each stage. It gives intervention a sense of direction. Certainly when someone is self-harming, and the overwhelming desire on the part of the carer is to stop them from doing it, knowing that they have some idea of how to go about it will give them the confidence to try.

References

Abraham, C. and Shanley, E. (1992). *Social Psychology for Nurses*. Edward Arnold, London.

Adam, K. S. (1985). Attempted suicide. *Psychiatric Clinics of North America*, **8**(2):183–202.

Ballinger, B. (1971). Minor self injury. *British Journal of Psychiatry*, **118**:535–8.

Brant, B. A. and Osgood, N. J. (1990). The suicidal patient in long term care institutions. *Journal of Gerontological Nursing*, **16**(2):15–18, 36–7.

Burrow, S. (1992). The deliberate self harming behaviour of patients within a British special hospital. *Journal of Advanced Nursing*, **17**:138–48.

Carr, E. G. (1977). The motivation of self injurious behaviour: a review of some hypotheses. *Psychological Bulletin*, **84**(4):800–16.

Courage, M. M., Godbey, K. L., Ingram, D. A., Schramm, L. L. and Hale, W. (1993). Suicide in the elderly: staying in control. *Journal of Psychosocial Nursing and Mental Health Services*, **31**(7):26–31.

Etzersdorfer, E. and Fischer, P. (1993). Suicide in the elderly in Austria. *International Journal of Geriatric Psychiatry*, **8**(9):727–30.

Evans, C. and Lacey, J. H. (1992). Multiple self-damaging behaviour among alcoholic women: a prevalence study. *British Journal of Psychiatry*, **161**:643–7.

Ferry, R. (1992). Self-injurious behaviours. *Senior Nurse*, **12**(6):21–5.

Hawton, K. and Fagg, J. (1992). Deliberate self poisoning and self-injury in adolescents: a study of characteristics and trends in Oxford. *British Journal of Psychiatry*, **161**: 816–23.

Hoff, L. (1989). *People in Crisis: Understanding and Helping*, 3rd edn. Addison-Wesley, Menlo Park, California.

Nowers, M. (1993). Deliberate self harm in the elderly: a survey of one London borough. *International Journal of Geriatric Psychiatry*, **8**(7):609–14.

Pederson, C. (1993). Promoting nursing students' positive attitudes towards providing care for suicidal patients. *Issues in Mental Health Nursing*, **14**(1):67–84.

Podvoll, E. M. (1969). Self mutilation within a hospital setting: a study of identity and social compliance. *British Journal of Medical Psychology*, **42**:213.

Reid, W. amd Long, A. (1993). The role of the nurse providing therapeutic care for the suicidal patient. *Journal of Advanced Nursing*, **18**:1369–76.

Ruthvern, A. M. (1987). Diagnosing self-harm in the elderly: a descriptive study. In *Classification of Nursing Diagnoses: Proceedings of the Seventh Conference held in St. Louis, Mo. 9–13 March 1986.* C. V. Mosby. St Louis, pp. 253–8.

Sonneborn, C. K. and Vamstraelen, P. M. (1992). A retrospective study of self-inflicted burns. *General Hospital Psychiatry*, **14**(6):404–7.

Stengel, E. (1964). *Suicide and Attempted Suicide*. Penguin, Harmondsworth.

van den Bent-Kelly, D. (1992). Too busy for trivia–patients who self harm. *Nursing: Journal of Clinical Practice, Education and Management*, **5**(5):32–3.

Suggested reading

Bellak, L., Abrams, D. M. and Ackermann-Engrel, R. (1992). *Handbook of intense brief and emergency psychotherapy (B.E.P.)*, 2nd edn. CPS Inc., Lanchmont, NY. (This North American text is designed for therapists working in crisis situations. It provides an excellent source of material for nurses wishing to explore their verbal interventions during PE.)

Long, K. A. (1986). Suicide intervention with Indian adolescent populations. *Issues in Mental Health Nursing*, **8**(3):247–53. (This is a particularly interesting case study dealing with the Wind River Reservation suicide epidemic in the American Northwest. Useful for considering alternative views of, and cultural obstacles to, self-harm.)

McLaughlin, C. (1994). Casualty nurses' attitudes to attempted suicide. *Journal of Advanced Nursing*, **20**(6):1111–18. (This paper explores the views of A&E staff in Northern Ireland towards the self-harming group.)

Valente, S. M. (1991). Deliberate self harm: management in a psychiatric setting. *Journal of Psychosocial Nursing and Mental Health Services*, **29**(12):19–25, 30–1. (Though not strictly about emergency situations it considers the problems faced by nurses in dealing with self-harm, and provides useful care strategies.)

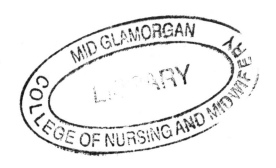

6

Threats of violence

Introduction

One of the most significant worries that nurses have is about threats of violence, either towards themselves or between their clients (Whittington and Wykes 1992). This is not restricted to mental health nurses. Over recent years the level of violence experienced by nurses in A&E departments has increased dramatically (Johnston 1987, Sheehan 1991), while those working with elderly clients have always had problems with apparently unprovoked attacks (Murray and Snyder 1991, Whall *et al.* 1992). On general medical and surgical wards too, violence precipitated by both medical conditions and patient frustration seems to be more common, and much of the work of liaison psychiatric nurses is spent counselling their general colleagues about this problem (Plylar 1989, Morrison 1993a). Nurses working in the community have always been at risk of violent attacks, but with the moves towards less institutional based care this risk will probably increase (Madela and Poggenpoel 1993).

Care developed for mental health clients places more emphasis upon their ability to cope with their own problems. Some of them simply do not want this type of care, and not all of them have either the ability or the professional support to be able to become involved successfully. The consequence has been an increase in reported violence from both residential and community-based nurses. A rise in the amount of wards being used solely for clients prone to violent activities, the prominence of specialist units for those clients with challenging behaviours and a general reduction in the amount of professional staff trained to work with those suffering from serious mental health problems, have all contributed to the current trend (Aiken 1984, Davis 1991, Caplan 1993). However, violence has always been a problem faced by healthcare workers.

Perhaps it is because nurses have to work with those people in society who are most vulnerable that they see a side to them which others do not. The pressure placed upon an individual entering hospital is enormous, and despite the possible support of friends and relatives, this pressure has to be borne on their own. The pain, discomfort and uncertainty of illness are all personal, while the circumstances in which they occur appear to the sufferer to be controlled by others. Those who care for those who are ill will always be held responsible for their recovery, and there are times when the care offered does not seem to match the care required. In a sense the failure of the patient to get well becomes the fault of the carer, and the frustration this engenders in the sick person has to be directed at someone. Usually it is the nurse, though of course, any professional offering direct contact may be a target. We must also add to this the psychological problems associated with the 'why me' syndrome, the downright unfairness of being the person who has to suffer, and the 'why couldn't it be someone else' syndrome, or 'there are others who deserve this more than me'. These too generate anger at the personal circumstances of the sufferer which again have to be directed at someone.

In a mental health setting this frustration may be the product of all of the above, but it can be exacerbated by the peculiarities of psychological disturbance. It is one thing to have to deal with the pressure of illness when you have access to your own logical thought processes, even if they are distorted by the personal nature of your suffering, but when these thoughts are also denied you, the situation becomes far more worrying. Not being able to make sense of where you are or what is happening to you, or making the wrong sense of everything and being confronted by the confusion this creates, are bound to increase your potential for violence. After all, most people become violent because they fear that they are in danger, either to their physical or psychological self. The vulnerability which mental disorientation brings can only increase their sense of insecurity, and violence may become the only course of action available to them (Meddaugh 1992).

The nature of violence

Violent behaviours are not restricted to absolute physical attacks. Aggression is a commodity which we all possess, and we use it to strengthen our resolve, especially in sporting and recreational activities. It acts as a driving force, motivating us to achieve higher levels of performance. Yet when we lose control over it, and it assumes a more sinister guise, it has the ability to make us antisocial and a threat to the safety of others. This is when aggression becomes violence. It is often measured in terms of the effects it has upon others; hence the fact that aggression usually causes offence and disturbance, while violence may induce fury and outrage, one inflicting anger, the other possibly injury.

People can be aggressive towards each other in simple ways, such as always making a point of being late for an appointment or never remembering another person's name. We tend to see this as rudeness. It can become more obvious in the sense that one individual always argues with another, or makes a point of disrupting another's plans. Such behaviour appears to be more conscious and disruptive, with one individual manipulating another. As the level of aggression increases so the effects it has on others also increases, often interfering with the victim's ability to control their own life. It may be a long and insidious process, or one of short outbursts, but it has the same disabling affect on those who bear the brunt of it. When violence does erupt it may or may not be foreseen, but it always has a cause. It may be as a result of the victim's losing patience with the aggressor, or the aggressor's wanting greater impact for their actions. Either way it will be forceful and disturbing for all those involved in it.

The violent behaviour can range from personal verbal abuse to full-blown physical assault. Once an individual has adopted a violent course of action there has to be a significant outcome. The purpose of aggression is to achieve a personal aim, be it self-protection or dominance over others, and this purpose has to be achieved at the expense of the victim. As violence occurs as a consequence of an increase in emotional pressure the aggressor may not be aware of the effect they are having upon others, and even less likely to know when to stop their actions. In some cases they cannot stop. For the victim of such outbursts, the suffering inflicted will be painful, either physically or emotionally, with the indignity of the whole episode being hard to cope with.

The motivation for such behaviour is sometimes relatively easy to discern, as in the case of someone who feels that an injustice is taking place and who wishes to put it right by attacking the perpetrator of the perceived crime. In other situations the cause may be far less obvious, and on occasions there appears to be no reason for the behaviour at all (Meddaugh 1992). However, there is always a reason. It is rare for violence to be totally without cause, and such behaviours are usually associated with people who have suffered head injuries or uncommon pathological conditions. Even then there will be a cause for the behaviour, but its nature is far more difficult and complex to diagnose.

Violence and the nurse

It seems something of an irony that nurses, in the pursuit of helping others, should find themselves the victims of all types of aggressive and violent acts, but the fact is that they do. This is not to suggest that each and every clinical situation is fraught with danger, that every patient or client is about to inflict some form of injury on the unsuspecting carer, or that all clients have to be viewed as potential attackers. The fact is that only a very small proportion of clients are ever likely to act in such a way, and that certain clinical environments are more prone to caring for them. However, such clients do not always present in these environments and the conditions for violence already discussed in this chapter may exist no matter where the client is.

Nurses need to be particularly mindful of the way they approach and interact with their client groups. Knowing that there are tremendous problems associated with being a client is of no value to the nurse if that knowledge is not taken into consideration when working with them. The nurse has to have an understanding of the nature of human behaviour, and not just the technical knowhow to implement care strategies or operate complicated therapeutic procedures. There has to be a balance between the art and science of nursing, which enables the nurse to combine human qualities in the pursuit of professional caring. Without such a balance the nurse is even more at risk of abuse, and may find that they are unable to deliver successful care.

One has to ask why it is that some nurses seem better able than others to deal with potentially violent and aggressive clients? Why is it that some nurses seem to be the victim of abuse more than others? Why do some clients always respond in a more violent way to some members of staff than others? There is no single answer to these questions, but there may be a common factor. Some nurses do not explore their own interpersonal behaviour enough to recognize that they have the potential to antagonize clients, while others are not aware of the effects they have on others. Such a lack of self-awareness is self-defeating within a care environment. Very rarely are the nurse's actions questioned following a violent incident. In most cases it is more likely that the client will be seen as being responsible, and their pre-morbid behaviour analysed and recorded. If the nurse is never seen as having some part to play in the development of such events, how can they hope to develop their skills in dealing more effectively with them in the future? Perhaps more significantly, why is it that the client is seen as the perpetrator? Is it because it is easier to blame someone for your own failings, and easier still to equate the mental health client with violence and aggression even though so few of them actually indulge in such extremes of behaviour. Whatever the reason, failure to explore the behaviours of all those involved in violent or aggressive events is both short sighted and therapeutically counter-productive.

It must not be assumed from the above that nurses are always responsible for untoward violent incidents. On the contrary, they are usually innocent victims, but it is true that many cases of violence by clients towards nurses could be predicted, even expected, if nurses do not use their observational and assessment skills correctly. Recognizing changes in behavioural patterns, identifying precipitants for such behaviours and learning when, and when not, to intervene with individual clients is one way of at least anticipating such events. This information can be used in an attempt to restore a client's emotional balance before s/he loses control or feels the need to become violent. Recognizing that an incident is imminent is almost as important as knowing what to do about it. It is certainly far less disturbing for all concerned to deal with a potentially violent situation than to have to deal with the actual event itself.

Preventing violence is not only less stressful, but, in theory at least, it should be more client-oriented. Once a client has become violent or aggressive it is almost impossible to reach them intellectually, to be able to reason with them, to ask them to use judgement and make considered decisions. In most cases the nurse will have to do all that for the client, to calm them in some way, and only afterwards get them to involve themselves in discussion about what might have been. If the nurse detects the immediacy of such an event, and acts before it gets out of hand, there is a greater possibility of involving the client in such problem-tackling activities, and, more possibility of their being in a state of mind to be able to benefit from them.

Violent and aggressive outbursts do not just happen, and are then forgotten about, they cause casualties. Not just people with physical pain, but those who have to try and get on with their lives irrespective of the abuse they may have suffered or inflicted. Both the attacker and the victim fall into this group, with no-one being immune from the sour aftermath of such events. Mixed emotions, hurt pride, unresolved personal differences, divided loyalties, loss of face, loss of dignity, all these, and many more besides, are the scars left behind after such outbursts. All these have to be dealt with before the process of caring can be continued, yet all too often there is neither the time, nor in some situations, the inclination, to do so. The consequence of this is that both client and nurse feel bitter about what took place and future interaction between them remains ineffective and sterile – hardly the basis for personal growth and development. While it is accepted that some incidents will take place, irrespective of the quality of supervision demonstrated by the nurse, prediction skills have to be developed if the unhelpful state of affairs described above is to be avoided.

Consider this analogy between earthquakes and violent incidents. A great deal is known about earthquakes, the effects they have and the consequences of their occurring. Over the years research has shown two things: how to predict when earthquakes are about to happen, and what to do to prepare yourself so that when they do take place damage is minimized. In areas prone to earthquakes, buildings are constructed so that they do not fall down so easily; nor are they built too high, in order to minimize devastation. When 'quakes are predicted the population has specific instructions about what to do to restrict the risk to life. The same applies to violent incidents. Knowledge of human behaviour has told us how to prepare against them and nursing theory gives us guidelines to minimize their effects. One further comparison exists within this analogy, in both cases prediction and preparation do not guarantee successful intervention.

Violence and AIRS

Violence may occur in any situation and in any number of guises. The nurse needs to be able to identify the potential for serious and harmful aggression within his/her working environment just as much as within the client group it involves. Nurses in accident and emergency departments are more likely to deal with such behaviours than, say, those within a maternity unit (Neades 1994), while those working with the elderly are often surprised at the extraordinarily high incidents of aggression that they are called upon to deal with (Ryden and Feldt 1992, Herz *et al.* 1992). Violent PEs cannot always be avoided but in many cases they can be predicted. Therefore, assessment of both the clinical environment as well as the client is of paramount importance. If there is a recognizable pattern associated with violence experienced within a particular area, strategies for dealing with it can be devised which, apart from giving staff a sense of confidence in planning for an event, also improve the organizational response to it. Fairlie and Brown (1994) have shown that it is possible to identify specific times of the day when such events may occur, and this simple study to examine accidents and incidents systematically over a six-month period could easily be replicated.

Assessment here also involves some form of analysis of staff performance in relation to violent incidents. While most authorities agree that all staff might, at some time or another, be involved in such events, those staff who seem less threatening or with a lower power base appear to attract less attention than their more power-conscious colleagues (Whittington and Wykes 1994). Morrison (1992) also identified feelings of intimidation and interpersonal control (coercion) as major contributory factors in aggressive incidents. These and other studies would suggest that nurses need to make sense of themselves just as much as they need to make sense of their clients.

It will be difficult for us to address these issues in any depth within this text, the main purpose of which is to identify what positive steps can be taken once this example of a PE has begun. However, selecting staff with a proven track record of effectiveness, good interpersonal skills, and an accommodating personal style in their approach to their practice may be the first step in the development of successful intervention strategies. Other personal and organizational skills are needed to intervene with any impact on a violent PE. We will explore these in more detail later in the chapter but in many ways they are similar in nature to those required when dealing with self-harming clients. In both cases, the motivation for the behaviour is aggression and in both cases the nurse has to respond, using the minimum of intervention to produce the maximum of response.

Resolution of an aggressive PE is difficult to describe. Most authors see the necessity to spend time with aggressive clients both during and after the event as crucial to its resolution but there are occasions when people want, and clearly need, to be left alone. The skill of the intervening nurse will be in determining how much contact is required and how safe is the alternative. A violent PE can be said to have been resolved only once the circumstances have been fully explored by the people involved. Assuming that all will be well after an aggressive outburst without finding out why it occurred, what effect it has and whether it is likely to reoccur, is both naive and dangerous.

Finally the necessity for support within a violent PE cannot be overstressed; feelings of anger and hurt associated with a personal attack within a clinical setting are akin to any experience by individuals within society who may or may not be attacked. The feelings of rejection, pain and helplessness can lead to individuals using behaviour out of keeping with professional nursing practice as well as those which may lead them to being attacked once more in the future. Over-compensating for a perceived 'softness' may lead to a nurse becoming hard and unapproachable, which in turn may be perceived as uncaring and combative by the client. Wandrak (1989) shows that most nursing students are verbally abused by clients within a mental health setting, yet they are often those with the least power and the least control within the clinical environment. They are, however, often the most vulnerable and consequently require the maximum supervision. Support is required both for this at-risk group and for everyone else involved, be they client or staff. Support should not be offered just to the point of resolution but should be forthcoming throughout the event where possible, during resolution and in the subsequent follow-up and analysis phase.

Support may be difficult to offer in certain cases such as in the situation where you are a junior member of staff and the charge nurse is the one who has been abused, but each member of staff should take responsibility for supporting each other. Of course, probably the most difficult person to support may be the client who has been responsible for the incident in the first place. It goes without saying that nurses will have to support this individual, though it can be stressful to have to spend time with a person who has just insulted you or physically attacked you. Procedures for handling this difficult scenario may be in place within a certain clinical area but it is something that needs to be addressed in detail before PEs of this nature occur. Nurses may be feeling too much stress or in too much pain to be able to become involved in the resolution or support phases of the PE. Who takes their place? If a procedure is not in place the likelihood is that it will be no-one in particular, with the likely eventuality being the resumption of the behaviour which precipitated the original aggressive incident. The consequences? More staff victims, more clients stressed and increasing potential for the use of medication to deal with problems that almost inevitably need people to sort them out.

Using AIRS as a guideline, what factors can be built in to our game plan, firstly to reduce the potential of aggressive PEs and secondly, deal with them effectively when they have occurred? We will concentrate on the following areas:

- predicting factors;
- client involvement;
- types of aggressive incidents;
- types of interventions;
- reaction times;
- support systems.

Predicting factors

Earlier in the chapter we considered the parallels between earthquakes and aggressive PEs. There is of course a major difference between predicting these two events. With the first, even if you predict correctly all you are able to do effectively is prepare yourself for the inevitable. With the latter, predicting may avert the event altogether. Can the aggressive PE be predicted? Most authors would say that they can. Like all forms of accurate prediction, it requires careful observation and the application of personal interaction skills. There are a number of variables which need to be considered when assessing the aggressive PE and authors vary in their identification and prioritization (Noble and Rogers 1989, Coldwell and Naismith 1989, Milius 1990). Morrison (1992) identifies four significant ones: a response to coercive behaviour, length of stay in hospital, a history of violence and specific clinical conditions, in particular Vipolar Affective Syndrome (VAS). From a nursing point of view these can be accommodated within the three critical components required for assessment.

1. Knowledge of the client's past history. This will include information about previous violent PEs, but also data concerning known precipitants to violence, precursors to the individuals violent behaviour and behaviour known to stimulate or exaggerate his or her anger.

2. Base line information about the client's behaviour is generally used to assess changes in mood.
3. Knowledge of human behaviour, to be able to assess the dynamic quality of interaction and its consequence. This includes both verbal and non-verbal behaviours, individual versus group performance and social exchange theories.

However, predicting is one thing, doing something with the prediction is another matter. A nurse may be extremely unpopular if, following a particularly unpleasant violent and aggressive incident, he/she tells their colleagues that they knew it was going to happen anyway! Consider this example:

> David is 23-years-old and very unhappy with both himself and life in general. He has been in the ward for a couple of days and his primary nurse has already noticed that there are times when David becomes irritable and intolerant of others. Usually this is later in the day, around early evening, and this has on one occasion led to a shouting match between David and an older male patient. The primary nurse documents this in David's profile but fails to stress its significance to other members of the team. A few days later when the primary nurse is off duty, David absconds from the ward and out on the street attacks a person who has asked him for directions.

What is significant here is not that the nurse was able to identify a key time in David's mood that was likely to favour the developments of an aggressive outburst but the method of communicating that information to his/her colleagues. It is of no value saying that it was written in the profile. Significant information has to be seen to be given significance. All those who might have been involved in David's care should have been aware of this crucial peak in the profile.

Client involvement

It will be reasonable to ask the question, 'How can you involve someone who has become so violent that he has actually lost control over his actions?' As already pointed out both in this chapter and in Chapter 1, if the client could control what s/he was doing, the PE would not take place. It is because of their lack of control that their behaviour has become so absolute. Therefore the question is not how, but when do you involve them?

Contemporary psychiatric nursing practice is based upon the therapeutic relationship between the client and nurse. This relationship has to be developed through mutual trust and co-operation with one offering time, skill and knowledge to help the other deal with their pain. This relationship can only work if there is a spirit of equality about it. That is not to say that both partners have to be equal in their skills etc.; that is patently not the case. The client needs the nurse's skill but also the nurse needs information from the client that only they can provide to be able to use that skill. The equality exists as a recognition of the work of the other for both partners. The equality, while recognizing successes and personal skills, also recognizes and accepts failings and deficiencies. Therefore if one partner makes a mistake, because they share a mutual relationship and trust each other's motives the mistake is just that – it is not an earth-shattering event. Likewise, if behaviours are used which are extreme or inappropriate, these too can be viewed differently within this relationship. It could be argued that this tolerance reduces the power differentials inherent in most professional relationships and therefore reduces the potential for violent and aggressive PEs.

However, if one occurs, and if the client has been used to being involved in decisions about his/her care then it follows that he/she ought to be involved in the decision which will determine how this is to be resolved. 'Talking people down', and 'being calm and talking in an even tone' are both examples of a description of the technique used to reduce the emotional explosion associated with an aggressive PE. They can be used as the link between the client's loss of control and their regaining it. Nonetheless, the process of giving responsibility to a client who is standing just a few inches from you, shouting and spitting in your face, is a difficult proposition to deal with. Inevitably unless the process of equality has existed before this event and the relationship has developed beforehand, it will be harder to manage the clients resumption of control. This is definitely not the time to start to develop such a relationship!

Clients need to be involved because involvement signifies worth and conveys self-esteem and dignity. The sooner the client can resume these feelings, the sooner he or she can begin to control the emotions associated with a PE. In a sense it is about taking responsibility for one's own actions or, in this case, about resuming responsibility. The nurse has to convey that he or she actually cares about the client and wants the best for him or her; this cannot be done by grappling somebody to the floor and holding them down every time they raise their voice or disagree with you. Similarly, clients who threaten and abuse regularly cannot be ignored on the basis that they are simply expressing themselves forthrightly. A balance needs to be struck between the client and the nurse within the framework of the relationship and based upon the client's therapeutic needs and the resources available to the nurse. Behavioural boundaries will be set agreeable to both parties with an acceptance of the consequences of stepping outside of those boundaries. If the client is unable to commit her/himself to such negotiations, either because their mental state precludes them or because they are not prepared to accept this form of personal responsibility, the nurse must decide how best to progress. In the case of those too disturbed the nurse has to act as if the agreement has been struck, giving both verbal and non verbal cues to his or her equality. If the client refuses to take part on the basis of conscious non-compliance, the nurse will need to construct a therapeutic programme for it to take place but begin it by starting at the point where the client is prepared to agree.

Types of aggressive PE

In earlier chapters we have seen that much of the PE literature deals with aggression and violence, yet not all PEs represent such a threat to others as do these. The incidents that will be dealt with in this and subsequent chapters are those which are the most common, i.e. verbal abuse, unprovoked attacks, or those from 'out of the blue', and attacks following confrontation. All of these have their own unique presenting features; however, we will use the example of verbal abuse as the framework through which to explore some of the other types.

Verbal abuse

Many may feel that being verbally abused has less personal consequences than being physically attacked, but this is certainly not always the case. For many nurses, being confronted by an aggressive individual shouting violently and insultingly at them is just as debilitating as being grabbed or struck. Yet, for some reason, many psychiatric nurses tend to disregard these events as merely being part of the job (Morrison 1993a). As a consequence, the clients are seldom given the opportunity to work through the reasons for the outburst while the nurses involved may receive, at most, a cursory 'You're OK, aren't you?' before the whole thing is forgotten about. The effects upon both client and nurse can be devastating and such flippancy is harmful and disorganizing.

Becoming desensitized to such behaviour may be the result of prolonged exposure to it, but doing nothing about it devalues the client's reasons for adopting such tactics and denies nurses access to support in dealing with professional and personal consequences. All PEs, no matter how minimal or spontaneous they may be viewed, must be treated in the same constructive way, with consideration being given to their causes and effects.

In cases of verbal abuse it is essential to explore the reasons for the outburst, the way that it was dealt with, and the support required for those involved after the events. It may take a client a long time to calm down afterwards, especially if it has been a particularly long and violent episode. Strategies for dealing with this emotional trauma have to be incorporated into the nurse's intervention. But other nurses must be aware of such approaches and sure that they follow the 'game plan'. In effect the PE may only last for a few violent seconds but the consequences can be felt for several hours afterwards. If not dealt with considerately the potential for further outbursts is dramatically increased.

As a general rule the most effective nursing approach to adopt in such situations involves passive response. It involves staying calm and demonstrating outwardly through passive body language that this is the case. Passive body language here includes not stepping forward, not stepping or moving toward the client, not raising your hands or voice, keeping out of the client's personal space, even sitting down where appropriate, and not staring straight into the client's eyes.

Several responses should be non-antagonistic with simple, unambiguous acknowledgements, such as 'Yes', 'I see', 'OK' etc. This is not the time to indulge the client in deep and meaningful counselling. The purpose of the response is to take the sting out of the emotional tension being expressed by the client and reduce the possibility of the event escalating into something more physically dangerous. Using empathetic responses such as 'You obviously feel very angry about this' or 'I can see how angry this is making you' can be useful here. They may sound strange things to say but surprisingly they have a deflating effect because they show the client that you are paying attention to the way he/she feels and not just what he/she is saying. They also give the impression of sharing the experience with the client rather than confronting them. Most importantly of all they give credence to the way he or she feels, in a way that gives permission for them to express their feelings. In doing so, the nurse becomes less of a target for attack; it also gives the nurse a breathing space while deciding what to say or do next. Certainly the client may respond in strange ways to such an approach but careful observation in such an interaction will reveal a lessening of the original force offered by the client and this is, after all, the desired effect of the initial interchange.

Consider again the example of David described earlier. This time, the primary nurse has paid special attention to the identified times when David was irritable and intolerant of others.

At about 6.00 p.m. the primary nurse began to pay particular attention to David, initially just being in his vicinity but gradually spending small amounts of time with him. The nurse knew that David, when verbally abusive, was loud, threatening and intimidating, and he had also established that David did not make physical contact and while expressing the desire to inflict harm, had never done so.

At 7.45 p.m. David was watching TV with another client and without warning suddenly leapt to his feet and began shouting, at first at the TV and then as a response to the other clients' insistence that he kept quiet. The nurse was only a few paces away and was soon separating the two individuals both of whom were well into a bout of abuse and threats. A second nurse joined them and began talking to the second client while the primary nurse concentrated on David. Having deflected his attention away from the other client by simply stepping between them and maintaining eye contact, the nurse's next task was to allow David the opportunity to vent his feelings without putting anyone in a dangerous position. Consequently, the nurse asked what had happened in a reasonable, quiet, expressionless tone of voice.

David's voice became even louder as he shouted obscenities at the nurse who only responded by a slight nod of the head. 'You are obviously very angry about something.' David's response was perhaps rather predictable: yes, of course he was angry, any fool could see that, what kind of a nurse did he think he was? etc. The nurse said nothing, nor did anything and kept his face as expressionless as possible and resisted looking straight into David's eyes. Feeling that the abuse had been redirected towards himself, the nurse next had to begin the task of diffusing it altogether. 'I don't like to see you so upset.' 'How can I help?' This took David by surprise and he obviously found it difficult to respond directly to this. 'What?' was all he could manage. The nurse repeated what he had said. David replied – and no longer in such a loud and aggressive way that nobody could help him – and indeed he didn't want anyone to help him because he didn't really need help.

Finally, the nurse moved to one side and sat down in the chair vacated by the other client and said, 'I must be able to do something, it doesn't seem fair that you should be so distressed.' Without thinking, David sat down beside him and, though still talking loudly, began to discuss the unfairness of his situation. Meanwhile the other nurse had carried a similar exercise with the other client about being the unwilling recipient of David's initial abuse. He had responded quickly to the nurse and agreed that the best thing to do for the time being was to move away from David. Other clients and visitors were generally reassured that all was well and no-one in any danger by the third member of the nursing team.

David spent about 30 minutes with the nurse and between them they agreed that they would talk the next day about issues that had arisen. David had admitted to feelings of frustration and irritability which he had attributed to boredom. They also agreed to meet at a time which coincided with an increase in the feelings, i.e. early evening, in an attempt to reduce them and any subsequent violent behaviour. The nurses had predicted that something might happen as well as the approximate time and the pattern of the disturbance. David's primary nurse had used this data to plan a strategy which meant that he could diffuse David's anger, while the others supported those who might be affected by the incident. After the event they spent a few minutes debriefing each other on their own actions and establishing that each of them had not been badly affected by the incident. The incident itself was fully documented for future reference at the nursing process review meeting. Particular attention was paid to the decisions that David and the nurse had made.

Types of intervention

Different forms of intervention are described during this and subsequent chapters, and the principles outlined in Chapter 4 apply here just as with any other PE. In this particular case the nurses were involved in non-physical direct contact, as is more likely to be the case in verbal abuse situations, though other techniques may sometimes need to be considered when the situation becomes a PE. While certain indirect interventions formed the basis of the nurse's work with David, several points can be made from this example:

1. The effective strategy for dealing with a potential episode had its roots in the observational work carried out beforehand. This was based upon the three criteria which determined that David was prone to verbal outbursts, did not offer physical violence, and was more likely to become abusive at a certain time of the day.
2. The use of an AIRS framework enabled the primary nurse to construct a strategy that had both a remedial effect but also a positive response to future events.
3. David was involved in decisions made about the event and as such took some responsibility for his own actions. The discussion with him that would follow would determine how much responsibility he was prepared to take and just what it was that he wanted to achieve once he had done so.
4. Because the team knew what to do in the event of an episode they were less likely to suffer harmful consequences at a later stage. The support required following the episode was minimal because of this preparation.

Some critics might make the observation that if nurses can predict the episodes likely to happen, it is unprofessional to allow them to take place. The answer to this is quite simply that you cannot assume anything is going to happen. If nurses make all the decisions for every client, remove stress factors, reshape their clinical environment and protect them from themselves, how can the client ever be expected to change their behaviour or take control of it? Clients have the right to make their own mistakes and nurses should be there to help the clients devise ways of dealing with them.

Reaction times

What is noticeable about this example is the response time of the nurse. With self-harming clients the actual response time to the client, i.e. the time taken to stop the behaviour from escalating, is often much longer even though the nurse might be in contact with the client. In the case of verbal abuse, the response time was very much shorter and once the nurse was on the scene he was trying to diffuse the situation from the very start of contact. The reactionary nature of the event means that any time spent not trying to reduce the emotional expression of the client may actually contribute to its increase. The difficulty for the nurse is trying to strike a balance between getting to the scene quickly and being able to control their own need to calm the client as quickly as possible. The reaction time is not about resolving the issue – that will have to take as long as it does – but about taking the sting out of the immediate burst of emotional energy expressed by the client. Some nurses are able to control themselves better than others, while some use techniques to calm themselves, like counting in their head in between responses to ensure that they do not seem too eager to impose on the client's thoughts.

Whatever method is employed, the secret is to remember that you cannot rush the resolution of this event. It has to run its course if it is to be dealt with effectively.

Support systems

Those who have been verbally abused will know that such situations can be just as humiliating and personally damaging as any other violent outburst against them. It is false to assume that nurses are able to deal with the trauma of personal abuse as if it had not happened. At the end of this book we will deal more fully with this issue, but just as AIRS requires support for clients in need, so too does it address the complex difficulties associated with staff support.

In incidents like the one involving David, perhaps the most supportive group available is the primary nursing team itself. Nurses working as a unit are more aware of the pressures placed upon their colleagues, because they are working with the same client group. However, support is needed both in terms of reassurance that others are there to discuss the event with, and also in a more formal sense as a debriefing for the event generally. This latter helps inform future intervention as much as supporting the individuals involved.

Conclusion

Verbal abuse is a difficult situation for nurses to deal with, not least because on the face of it such things are seen as relatively harmless in the overall pattern of nursing. This may, or may not be true, but I suspect that for those who have been violently abused there is little distinction between any form of abuse. It is essential that the nurse feels supported by their own knowledge of the situation, of the client, of the intervention and the outcomes that might be anticipated. The example used in this chapter highlighted these key issues, and as such raised questions about predicting and preparing for such outbursts.

While it is not always possible to detect the potential for a violent outburst or PE, it can be done. However, what prediction should give the nurse is the ability to plan an effective strategy for dealing with the event if it does take place; a plan which promotes client involvement in a satisfactory resolution, reduces the risk of escalation beyond verbal interchanges, and ultimately provides the nurse with the confidence to implement the plan.

References

Aiken, G. J. M. (1984). Assaults on staff in a locked ward: prediction and consequences. *Medicine, Science and the Law*, **24**:199-207.

Caplan, C. (1993). Nursing staff and patient perceptions of the ward atmosphere in a maximum security forensic hospital. *Archives of Psychiatric Nursing*, 7(1):23–9.

Coldwell, J. B. and Naismith, L. J. (1989). Violent incidents on special care wards in a special hospital. *Medicine Science and the Law*, **29**(2):116–23.

Davis, S. (1991). Violence by psychiatric inpatients: a review. *Hospital and Community Psychiatry,* **42**:585–90.

Fairlie, A. and Brown, R. (1994). Accidents and incidents involving patients in a mental health service. *Journal of Advanced Nursing,* **19**:864–9.

Herz, L. R., Volicer, L., Ross, V. and Rheaume, Y. (1992). A single case-study method for treating resistiveness in patients with Alzheimer's Disease. *Hospital and Community Psychiatry,* **43**(7):720–4.

Johnston, J. B. (1987). Violence in the emergency department. *Emergency Nursing Reports,* **1**(12):1–7.

Madela, E. N. and Poggenpoel, M. (1993). The experience of a community characterized by violence: implications for nursing. *Journal of Advanced Nursing,* **18**(5):691–700.

Meddaugh, D. I. (1992). Lack of privacy control may trigger aggressive behaviours. *Provider,* **18**(7):39.

Milius, A. C. (1990). Experienced psychiatric nurse's predictions of in-patient aggression. *Kansas Nurse,* **65**(10):10– 11.

Morrison, E. F. (1992). A coercive interactional style as an antecedent to aggression in psychiatric patients. *Research in Nursing and Health,* **15**(6):421–31.

Morrison, E. F. (1993a). The measurement of aggression and violence in hospitalized psychiatric patients. *International Journal of Nursing Studies,* **30**(1):51–64.

Morrison, E. F. (1993b). A comparison of perceptions of aggression and violence by psychiatric nurses. *International Journal of Nursing Studies,* **30**(3):261–8.

Murray, M. G. and Snyder, J. C. (1991). When staff are assaulted: a nursing consultation service. *Journal of Psychosocial Nursing and Mental Health Services,* **29**(7):24–9, 39–40.

Neades, B. L. (1994). How to handle aggression. *Emergency Nurse,* **2**(2):21–4.

Noble, P. and Rodgers, S. (1989). Violence by psychiatric inpatients. *British Journal of Psychiatry,* **155**:384–90.

Plylar, P. A. (1989). Management of the aggressive head injury patient in an acute hospital setting. *Journal of Neuroscience Nursing,* **21**(6):353–6.

Ryden, M. B. and Feldt, K. S. (1992). Goal directed care: caring for aggressive nursing home residents with dementia. *Journal of Gerontological Nursing,* **8**(11):35–42.

Sheehan, A. (1991). RMNs have a part to play: mental health nurses within A&E facilities. *Nursing,* **4**(37):8.

Wandrak, R. (1989). Dealing with verbal abuse. *Nurse Education Today,* **9**(4):276–80.

Whall, A. L., Gillis, G. L., Yankou, D., Booth, D. E. and Beel-Bates, C. A. (1992). Disruptive behaviour in elderly nursing home residents: a survey of nursing staff. *Journal of Gerontological Nursing*, **18**(10):13–17.

Whittington, R. and Wykes, T. (1992). Staff strain and social support in a psychiatric hospital following assault by a patient. *Journal of Advanced Nursing*, **17**(4):480–6.

Whittington, R. and Wykes, T. (1994). Violence in psychiatric hospitals: are certain staff prone to be assaulted? *Journal of Advanced Nursing*, **19**:219–25.

Suggested reading

Gluck, M. (1981). Learning a therapeutic verbal response to anger. *Journal of Psychosocial Nursing and Mental Health Services*, **19**(3):9–12. (Discusses personal styles of response to aggressive verbal behaviour and recommends the use of a well-planned approach.)

Smith, M. E. and Hart, G. (1994). Nurses' responses to patient anger: from disconnecting to connecting. *Journal of Advanced Nursing*, **20**:643–51. (This paper attempts to identify the events that lead up to the decisions made by nurses about what to do in difficult aggressive PEs.)

Morrison, E. F. (1994). The evolution of a concept: aggression and violence in psychiatric settings. *Archives of Psychiatric Nursing*, **8**(4):245–53. (Provides information on intervention styles based upon empirical evidence from the author's extensive research.)

7

Physical attacks

Introduction

As we have seen in Chapter 6 verbal abuse is a serious problem
for all nurses, but of course not all aggressive PEs are restricted
to verbal exchanges. The threat of a physical attack in nursing
is a very real one, with those working in certain specialities such
as A&E, care of the elderly, community care and mental health,
being particularly at risk (Johnston 1987, Department of
Health Advisory Committee 1988). However, the nature of a
physical attack can be as varied as one person pushing another
aside to one which involves weapons and places individuals at
risk of losing their lives. Physical attacks, as PEs, tend to be
situations where nurses are placed in dangerous situations by
clients attempting to reduce the perceived threat of danger to
themselves. They tend to fall into three separate categories:

1. attacks 'out of the blue' or unprovoked;
2. attacks following confrontation;
3. attacks motivated by the client's mental state which may
   also be a combination of items 1 and 2.

This text is concerned with all of these. It is less concerned
with those factors precipitating violent incidents and more with
what to do when they occur. The PE which involves a personal
attack either towards the nurse, the visitor or another client, is
one where the principal of speedy response is most characterized.
We will explore two situations using the framework identified
for the verbal abuse PE of Chapter 6 to see how techniques for

reducing the emotional tension and, in this case, speeding up the resolution time, can be incorporated into the nurse's game plan.

Issues relating to the third category, the client's mental state, are discussed in more detail in Chapter 10.

The unprovoked attack

Most violent PEs usually show signs of the impending event (Jones and Littler 1992). However, even if the nurse fails to recognize the cues being given out by the client or because the nurse walked straight into a situation 'cold', there are occasions when the violent PE seems to occur without warning. At such times it is essential that the nurse extricates him/herself from the attack as soon as possible while seeking an opportunity to provide positive support to the client. There are no rules to guard the nurse and in most cases this is the most difficult of the PEs for nurses to deal with because of its unexpected nature. Can AIRS help? In this case AIRS can only be used once the PE has begun, which makes the assessment very subjective and the intervention responsive, thus leaving the resolution and support as the only planned part of the framework. This should not deter the nurse from using AIRS. Experienced nurses will be better equipped to assess which situations might potentially lead to unprovoked attacks, though all nurses should be aware of danger signals, be they environmental, such as going into someone's home or a building that they are unfamiliar with; sociological, being on their own or unsupported; biological, being physically tired or unprepared for work; or psychological, not concentrating and being mentally unprepared to work with a particular client, or feeling that they do not have the abilities to work with a threatening client. Some nurses might also add a fifth dimension, that of emotional signals, where the nurse is unhappy about working with factors from any one of the other four and/or feels rejected by the client.

The purpose of intervention

While the nurse will obviously strive to be ready for any eventuality, it is not possible to be alert and vigilant the whole time.

Simple distractions, pressure of work, concentrating on other priorities and human error may all play a part. From a client's perspective, changes in mood, increases or alterations in symptoms, feelings and responses to those symptoms, levels of stress and perception of danger all may precipitate violent behaviour. So, once the nurse finds him/herself involved in an unprovoked attack, they are less likely to be able to resolve it as effectively as one which they had predicted. Therefore, nurses must reduce their initial expectation of the impact that they may have on the PE, aiming primarily to remove the threat to themselves or others (Cahill *et al.* 1991). Only then can they seek to identify the root cause of the outburst and follow it through, using some form of crisis intervention strategy. Consider the following example:

Julie is a psychiatric nurse working in the community. She has been working with Patricia for about six months following the latter's discharge from a hostel for the long-term mentally ill. On average, Julie spends about four hours a week with Patricia and they have been working on a variety of issues all designed to deal with difficulties Patricia faces returning to the community. The two have always got on well, having known each other prior to the outreach programme. For the last few weeks Patricia has become increasingly distressed about her relationship with her elderly parents. They live about a mile away but refuse to communicate with her, having not made contact for several years. As Patricia progresses through her rehabilitation programme, she is finding it difficult to cope with this apparent rejection. Last week, Patricia felt that it would be a good idea to write to her parents. She did so with Julie's encouragement and the last time Julie saw her was still awaiting a reply. This will be the fifth visit since the letter was sent.

As Julie stood at the door she felt something was not quite right, usually Patricia was waiting for her, but today she had already knocked twice and there was no reply. She decided to go around to the back of the house and turned to walk back down the path. As she did so, the front door flew open and Patricia came running out, ran straight at Julie and knocked her to the floor. She was shouting and crying at the same time and started beating her fists on Julie's shoulder. Julie was not hurt but she was taken aback and she was at a disadvantage being on the floor with a very stressed Patricia standing over her hitting her from behind. She tried to get up but this only made Patricia more angry, she began trying to kick out at Julie shouting, 'It's your fault.'

Julie managed to move around so that she was facing Patricia and said in a loud voice, 'Please stop doing this, Patricia, you are hurting me.'

'You deserve it.' Patricia again tried to kick out at Julie but because she was now facing her, Julie was able to move out of the way. In doing so, she put some small distance between the two of them and sprang to her feet. 'Please, Patricia, don't hurt me, please tell me why you are so upset.' Patricia was beginning to cry even more but was still trying to hit out at Julie who in turn was moving slowly backwards out of arm's reach. If necessary she was going to put the garden gate between the two of them but had already sensed that the attack was diminishing. 'What is it that I have done to offend you in such a terrible way?' she asked. Patricia, now sobbing almost uncontrollably, just turned and ran back into the house and slammed the door behind her. The PE was over. Now Julie had to find a way to resolve the situation.

The attack was violent and short-lived as is often the case. Julie was not badly hurt though she was bruised and distressed by the event. This is partly because of the physical violence but also because of the absolute rejection she felt from Patricia, a person with whom she had developed a good professional relationship. What can we learn from this example?

1. Immediate response

Julie's response was instant. She had no choice: she was a victim and the attack came from behind. She knew something was not quite right and perhaps she should not have turned her back on the front door, till she was a few paces away from the house. However, once she was attacked she responded positively in two ways. One, to protect herself, two, to set up a simple dialogue with Patricia.

2. Protection

Julie protected herself by facing Patricia and getting up as soon as she could. She then stayed out of arm's reach, always facing towards Patricia. She did not turn her back again, but kept moving backwards towards the gate.

3. Simple dialogue

As she got her breath back, recovering from the initial attack, she tried to distract Patricia by asking her questions but also by appealing to her conscience. 'Please do not hurt me,' she said, thus putting the responsibility on to Patricia to stop but not offering a threat as a response to the violence. The words and phrases used were unambiguous and uncomplicated.

4. Non-threatening response

Julie did not threaten Patricia with a punitive response. At no time did she offer violence herself but made it difficult for Patricia to maintain her aggressive posture by reducing the response to seeking answers to some simple questions. She did not 'stand up' to Patricia by offering violence. Such a move would have made the resolution of the PE even more difficult. Don't forget that Julie has to work with Patricia, not just to resolve this situation, but for a long time to come. Offering violence would destroy any trust that Patricia has for Julie. 'No confrontation' was therefore her game plan.

5. Quick assessment

During the first few seconds of the attack, Julie was working out how best to extricate herself from danger and planning ahead as to how to do it. She was not trying to work out what was the cause of the attack though she probably could have guessed. This would come later during the resolution phase.

6. Making a plan

Julie decided on a course of action. By doing so it gave her a specific purpose and in doing so enabled her to regain her poise. The plan was simple: keep talking and retreat and get the gate between the two of them. As it was she did not need to go that far but the knowledge that she had a plan gave her the confidence to carry on acting in a controlled and effective way.

7. No physical contact

Despite Patricia's trying to hit out at Julie at no time did Julie try to grab at Patricia or try to restrain her in any way. Julie did not take responsibility for Patricia's behaviour and allowed Patricia the dignity of stopping the aggression of her own accord. Restraint would have shifted the balance of power to Julie and Patricia would have stopped because Julie coerced her into doing so. Constraint was obviously inappropriate in this case, for the reasons discussed already, and dangerous because had Julie been unable to contain Patricia, Julie had no-one to support her and she could well have suffered an even more serious attack as a consequence.

8. No heroes!

All of Julie's behaviour was designed to get herself out of danger. She would not stand up to Patricia, threaten, or confront her. She did not try to coerce her into stopping the attack. However, she did keep out of arm's reach and backed away, albeit in a controlled fashion. In doing so, she did not pose a threat to Patricia, retained her professional countenance and dignity, and was able to stop the attack by staying calm. Eventually, Patrica had nothing to fight against. The key points to remember are:

1. make an immediate response;
2. protect yourself (or the individual being attacked);
3. start a simple dialogue;
4. use a non-threatening response;
5. carry out a quick assessment;
6. make a plan;
7. do not make physical contact;
8. do not be a hero.

Then, carry out the resolution and support phases of AIRS.

An assault following confrontation

As we have seen, most aggressive PEs can be predicted and certainly the changes that take place in the client's behaviour prior to such events should give enough warning to the nurse to modify their approach or take evasive action. The behaviours often described by authors are in the class of fight or flight responses generated by the autonomic nervous system coupled with certain behavioural changes. It is worth remembering that such things as 'the pupils becoming dilated', or the breathing becoming rapid and shallow, often quoted as biological changes prompted by feelings of anger, may be significant but they are often very difficult to detect in an emergency. Most nurses are more likely to see a combination of nervous system responses and behavioural changes. Neades (1994) highlights eight main features which describe posture, voice changes, attitude and behaviour. She also points out that any one of these may appear and they may appear in any combination. It is only during the PE – that part of a behavioural continuum where everything becomes extreme – that the nurse may actually be able to detect the potential for aggression and violence. Behaviours which might indicate an aggressive PE are:

- tense, agitated behaviour, pacing up and down, being unable to sit down, not able to continue a conversation or concentrate on anything for more than a few moments;
- the voice becoming louder and the pitch going up; shouting does not always follow but obviously when it has got to that level the PE has probably already begun;
- responding to others in an abrupt and possibly abusive manner;
- the pupils of the eyes become dilated, the face may become reddened, breathing increases and the skin appears moist and clammy;
- facial grimacing may occur as a consequence of the increased muscle tension;
- hands may be made into a fist opening and closing;
- the client may knock things over with the fist, hit inanimate objects or punch the palm of the other hand;
- responses may be sarcastic or abusive; obscenities may be used especially towards staff.

In situations where such behaviours are evident the nurse will need to respond in a planned and co-ordinated fashion if no-one is to get hurt or the PE is to be averted.

Smith and Hart (1994), in a Canadian survey of nurses' perceptions of anger, showed that when the threat of violence was perceived as high, then the nurses in the survey were inclined to disconnect, or withdraw from the client, but as the threat of violence reduced the nurses were more prepared to try to connect, or spend time with, the client. This is an interesting conclusion and one that is common within the literature on the subject (Gluck 1981, Podrasky and Sexton 1988, Turnbull *et al.* 1990). Bandura (1982) suggested that as we are presented with higher levels of stress, anger or threats to self, our confidence in our ability to deal with it reduces. Nurse self-efficacy is a key issue in the successful resolution of a predicted aggressive PE. More importantly one has to consider that a PE which follows confrontation between a client and a nurse will probably have occurred because the nurse was confident in their approach and felt able to deal with the consequences. If, as the literature suggests, nurses would prefer to withdraw from an aggressive PE if they feel threatened, on the basis that they feel they cannot deal effectively with it, then one has to ask the question, are they also aware of these inabilities while challenging the client in the first place?

The answer is not a simple one. Several factors, such as the nature of the client/nurse relationship, the client's mental state, the nature of the confrontation etc., all have to be considered. However, what is clear is that the more threatening the PE is to the nurse, the more difficult it becomes to make decisions about how to deal with it. Smith and Hart describe this scenario in terms of personalizing the aggression. The greater the threat, the more personal the event becomes, and the more the nurse questions their self-efficacy.

The nursing approach

The 'threat–self-doubt' cycle is difficult to break out of unless the nurse is aware of the effects of their actions upon others, has developed skills in interpersonal effectiveness, feels supported in their clinical actions, has confidence to deal with the situation for which they must take responsibility, and last but not least, has a definite plan of action which can be used when they appear to be losing influence over a situation. If the nurse has good insight into their own response to perceived threats of violence as well as insight into the behavioural presentation that precipitates such events and can combine these with a practical sense of what can be achieved, then it is likely that predicted aggressive PEs can be dealt with effectively. What nurses have to overcome is the dissonance associated with a failure in one of these three crucial components.

In the case of an assault following a confrontation this would mean, firstly, the nurse understanding the effects that the confrontation might have upon the client, including insight into their own performance, either as the confronting nurse or as a member of the team supporting that nurse. Secondly, the ability to recognize when the confrontation has generated anger in the client and the level of aggressive response that it is generating. Thirdly, to have a game plan for directing the aggression away from the assaulting process into something constructive, such as the resolution of the problem that generated the confrontation in the first place. At the very least, this game plan must be designed to reduce the sense of threat perceived by the nurse, thus increasing their potential to deal with it confidently and competently.

AIRS and the confrontational assault

A confrontation can be any situation where two or more individuals argue about the rightness of a particular subject or event. In nursing terms, most confrontational assaults arise as a result of clients and nurses disagreeing about care styles, progress, personal freedom and control issues. In mental health they may also occur as a consequence of the clients' disturbance or an increase in symptoms, and as a direct result of certain irrational thoughts and beliefs both about themselves and others.

In some cases confrontation may begin with a simple disagreement which may lead to an argument and escalate to some form of assault. In other cases it may be part of an antagonistic sequence of interaction brought about by the client's reaction to his or her condition or problems. It must also be said that some clients are significantly more aggressive than others and use confrontation as a way of asserting themselves. Either way, prior knowledge of the client's baseline behaviour is fundamental to any assessment of his/her current state of mind. If this assessment tells the nurse an aggressive incident is likely then the intervention between nurse and client must be altered accordingly, to reduce the conflict or the possibility of it. Where this is not possible, either because the client is losing control of their emotional self too rapidly, or because they have decided to use force to get what they want, the use of predetermined interventions designed to reduce the impact of the aggressive outburst is called for.

The resolution of this particular form of PE will occur once the client has regained control and/or is able to limit the emotional response to their feelings so that they can discuss the issue more appropriately. Support, both for the client and the nurse is continuous through these first three elements with the nurse providing support for the client before, during and after the event, and other members of staff supporting the nurse in a similar fashion. Of course AIRS can be used as a simple template for the assaultive PE but there are bound to be constraints placed upon its use. The nurse undertaking the assessment may not have the self-confidence to deal with the results of the confrontation, in which case he/she should know when to seek help or advice before the situation gets out of control, not once it has done so. The nurse is just as likely to be the cause of the PE as any other precipitant and the possibility increases as the nurse becomes less capable of handling the effects of his/her actions. Nurses should seek supervision from their colleagues, when dealing with difficult-to-handle or potentially violent situations or clients.

Interventions may have been predetermined but may be inappropriate once the PE occurs and nurses will have to 'make it up' as they go along. In truth, 'make it up' is not as spontaneous as it sounds. A nursing team should have carefully considered outcome measures to help them deal with this and any other PE. These measures should be based upon certain key philosophical as well as practical issues which will include: how the client is to be handled, who should carry out the intervention, who will take responsibility, and the client's role in the resolution phase. In most cases these issues will dictate the nature of the interaction; hence, 'make it up' is essentially a form of modification rather than one of creativity.

Resolution may be extremely difficult to define and describe in such situations. Certainly having a plan to deal with these eventualities, either as a standard practice procedure or specifically designed for a particular client, will provide a certain confidence in the efficacy of the care approach. In turn, this may reflect back upon the performance of the individual nurses involved and give them an indication of both the purpose of the interventions and knowledge about its settlement. Of course, things do not always go to plan. Consequently, there is no way of knowing how long the intervention will take before it is effective, and certainly time factors should not be written into such strategies. Resolutions will occur once the danger of the flashpoint of PE have passed but, here again, care needs to be taken that the intervention itself does not act to sustain the level of aggression. Grabbing hold of a client who is attempting to hit a nurse may be an effective way of ensuring that the nurse does not get hurt but what do you do once you have grabbed hold? When do you let go? How long must you hold on before the client says, 'OK, sorry, I made a mistake'? It is just as likely that grabbing hold will sustain the client's anger and that he or she will do what they can to break the hold and continue with their chosen course of action.

Similarly, if a nurse has been hit or hurt or is in pain following an assault, often the last thing they want to do is to help the individual who has just inflicted the injury. It is easy to say that as a nurse it is part of the job and one should put one's feelings to one side to help the client; it is another actually to be there having been frightened, abused and assaulted by a person who appears to care little or nothing for you, despite the fact that you are attempting to help them and be expected to use your skills and personal technology to help them get over the situation.

In some cases the nurses may remain in danger until they can be helped by others. In these situations resolution may only occur when those others arrive and all the nurse can hope to do is to reduce the potential for further assault by attempting to remain calm, not offering resistance and reducing the confrontational elements of their interactions with the client. Of course in some situations, the most obvious thing to do is shout out for help and keep on shouting until it arrives. Nurses might find themselves getting out of the client's way rather than getting in it as the best method of dealing with the assault, and in extreme cases, locking oneself in the toilet or putting something between yourself and the client while attempting to draw the attention of colleagues might be the most effective thing that can be done.

However, resolution still has to occur with the least possible harm coming to those involved in the assault. Resolution, no matter what the contingency plans or intervention used, will occur only when the flashpoint has passed and not, as might be considered the case, when the situation has been dealt with fully with the antecedents being carefully considered and dealt with. Resolution will constitute the end of the assault not necessarily the end of the aggression.

Support offered to both the client and the nurse will be determined by such things as resources, procedures and care programmes. However, it is essential that as an absolute minimum a client who has been assaulted, or who has carried out an assault, must not be left alone following the event, no matter how this is to be undertaken, and nurses who have been assaulted are not left to sort out the situation for themselves. Simply saying to a nurse who has been assaulted, 'Are you OK?' and expecting an honest and complete answer is foolish. Nurses need time to recover from such situations and the minimum they should expect is time out to begin the process. Another nurse ought to take over the responsibility of staying with the client following a PE but that may not always be possible. Though desirable, it may also not always be possible for nurses to be debriefed as soon as the event has occurred. Resources on a ward or in the community, or wherever the event may take place, may restrict the support process but it is the responsibility of every colleague to ensure that their team members are not left unsupported at such times.

Nurses who have been assaulted often feel abused and humiliated, and it would be nonsensical to expect them to function after such an event as if nothing had happened irrespective of their grade, seniority or experience. Clients may only have begun the process of showing how they feel. After all, the assault was carried out for a purpose and they are going to need support in dealing with their own feelings both about the assault and its intentions.

Let us consider some of these issues in the following example of an assaultive PE which occurred after the nurse, Sally, had been asked to talk to Janet about the noise she was making in her room. In this particular case, Sally was not Janet's primary nurse nor was she a member of Janet's care group. It was intended as a simple request to turn down the volume on a radio.

Sally knocked upon Janet's door in the hostel ward and got no reply. She knocked once again. Still no reply. She could hear the radio playing music loudly in the room and assumed that Janet could not hear her. She knocked once more and slowly opened the door, stepped into the room and discovered that Janet was not there. She moved over to the radio and turned the volume down. As she was turning to leave, Janet appeared in the doorway and asked her what she was doing. Sally explained what had happened and moved to leave the room. Janet said that she did not want to turn the radio down because she could not hear it when she was sitting out in the hallway. Sally suggested that she take the radio with her or sit in her room to listen to it. Janet complained that she could not listen to it in the hallway because there was no socket. Sally said that she would either have to leave the door open or sit in her room. She also asked if there was not somewhere else that Janet could go so that she could listen to the radio.

Up until this point Janet had remained reasonably calm about the whole thing. However, she began to raise her voice. Why, she wanted to know, did she have to move and why was it always her that had to do what others wanted; why were her wishes not taken into her consideration? Sally was not prepared for this; she did not know Janet very well, but did know that she could become aggressive if she were made to change her routines or carry out activities that she did not really want to do. Sally answered as best she could, that it was a communal building and that each person had to take some responsibility for what happened within it. She said that she was not personally aware of others imposing on Janet but would ask other members of staff for some clarification. She also said that she was not trying to stop Janet from doing what she wanted but was just trying to ensure that she looked after the interests of all the residents. Janet's voice became louder as she accused Sally of being a liar. She had, she said, been stopped from doing numerous things recently and cited a couple of examples. She also moved towards

Sally and was only a few paces from her. Sally could not get out of the room without moving past Janet who was effectively blocking her exit.

Sally asked Janet what ideas she had to try and sort out the problem. Janet however only became angrier at this suggestion, telling Sally that she should have asked her opinion in the first place instead of trying to 'Lord it over her'. Sally apologized for not thinking of this herself and pointed out that she had only tried to turn the volume down because Janet was not in the room herself. She asked if they could sit down and talk about it; however, by now Janet was standing directly in front of Sally and was becoming very angry. She was puffing her cheeks in and out, clenching her fists and breathing quite rapidly. Sally knew that they were approaching a flashpoint and decided to get out of the way as best she could. OK, she said, we can talk about this later. So saying, she stepped to one side and made towards the door. As she did so, Janet slapped her hard across the side of her face and shouted out that she was a liar and a cheat. She turned to face her and was trying to hit her again but Sally had covered her face with her hands and was moving backwards away from her.

Janet moved forward and was shouting loudly that Sally was not going to get away with it and as she swung at Sally with her hands, Sally leapt over the bed effectively placing the bed between the two of them and allowing her to move backwards unhindered through the door. Janet was slow to move around the bed to follow and Sally stood in the doorway holding her injured face which by now had started to sting badly. Sally was aware of someone coming up behind her, turned and saw another member of staff joining her. He asked what was happening but before Sally could answer, Janet started shouting that she was a liar and a cheat and that she had wanted to lock her up and steal her radio. The second nurse moved Sally to one side and stood between her and Janet, effectively reducing the possibility of a further assault on her. New to the situation, he was calmer and more controlled and perhaps more significantly knew Janet well. He had dealt with these outbursts before and he told Janet that she looked very upset and he was concerned about her. He suggested that they step into the hallway where there was more room to move about and invited Janet to help him sort the problem out.

Feeling that Janet was beginning to calm down with this new approach, he asked Sally if she would do something for him elsewhere in the hostel, thus getting Sally away from the incident, but in a position to provide support if necessary. Because a series of empathetic and responsive replies to Janet's demands were used, the emotional situation was diffused within a couple of minutes. The nurse spent some time with Janet talking about issues related to hostel life and they agreed to talk about the incident again later in the day. Most importantly the nurse made sure that Janet was aware that she had assaulted Sally and that such behaviour was not acceptable, nor was it likely to get Janet what she wanted. It was agreed that Sally and Janet, with the second nurse acting as an arbitrator, would need to talk about the situation once things had calmed down.

In this example the nurse behaved as most people would in everyday circumstances. However, these were not everyday circumstances. She did not know the client very well, she entered the room uninvited, she touched the client's property without asking, and placed herself in a dangerous position inside the room without giving thought to how she would get out of it. Not until she was confronted by a client showing the classic behavioural presentation of a potentially aggressive PE did she begin to use her professional skills, and by that time it was already too late. Only after she had been struck by the client did she demonstrate an awareness of what she was doing, and it was perhaps fortunate for her that the second nurse came to her assistance.

Nurses are always going to work with clients that they do not know very well, or who are new to them. Simple rules of politeness and courtesy apply to these interactions in just the same way as they should to any other. Clients who appear to be disempowered by nurses are more likely to become angry. Unfortunately those clients are often wrongly accused of having provoked the PE, when in fact that responsibility is more the domain of an inept, or impolite, nurse. Consider the above example within another context, say that of an average home. A teenage daughter has her radio playing loudly in her room. Other members of the household complain and eventually mother goes into the girl's room and turns the radio down – daughter shouts at mother that she has no privacy, and proceeds to give everyone in the house a hard time. Daughter is seen as a problem, but is she? Could there be some truth in her accusations, and are they likely to be ignored? The next day at school she tells her friends that life at home is unfair, and her friends agree with her!

In some respects the offhand way that some nurses respond to their clients can be seen as similar to the parent–child example above. However, when mothers and daughters argue, they rarely become physically violent towards each other because of the relationships that exist between them. For clients and nurses this relationship does not exist, or may only be in the early stages of development, and therefore there are fewer constraints placed upon the client in responding to what they see as threats to their dignity, self-respect or even physical safety.

The nurse, Sally, should not have entered the room once she discovered that the client, Janet, was not in it. She should have sought her out and discussed the volume of the radio in a less formal, parental, way. She may still have had difficulty getting Janet to respond appropriately, but at least she would not have been trapped in a room having been assaulted once, with further assault quite possible.

What did the nurse do that was right? She recognized the behavioural signs of impending aggression that Janet displayed, and when she realized that she was in a dangerous environment, and unlikely to be able to defend herself effectively, she tried to disconnect from Janet as quickly as she could. Even though she had been assaulted she managed to avert any further attack by jumping over the bed and getting into the doorway of the room. She remained with Janet even though the PE had still not yet been resolved. At no time did she respond to Janet's aggression with an aggressive response of her own.

If we combine the actions the nurse carried out that were appropriate, with those she could have used as an alternative, we finish up with these points.

- The nurse should never place herself at risk. Escape routes should always be available.
- Behaviour should not be used which demeans the client in some way. Personal property should always be respected.
- Politeness and co-operation are essential within the interaction.
- The client's wishes should be sought, before, not after, suggesting alternatives.
- The nurse must be aware of client behavioural changes indicating the potential for a violent response.
- Every attempt should be made to remain calm.
- The nurse should not respond violently to client aggression.
- The nurse should manoeuvre so that something is between the client and themselves.
- When in danger, the nurse should get out of it as quickly as possible.
- The nurse must not leave the client unattended following the event.
- Following the event, support for both the client and the nurse is essential.

• The PE is only resolved when the threat of immediate violence has diminished.

The second nurse's response to the PE is also quite interesting here. When he arrived he recognized that the nurse was in danger, and realized that she had been struck. He placed himself between the nurse and the client, and, instead of talking directly to the nurse, thus excluding the client, he talked to the client. He knew the client better than the first nurse, and had dealt with this type of situation before. Despite this he did not enter the room, and remained at a distance from the client as he spoke to her. As he had not been affected by the initial attack in the same way that the first nurse had, he was in a better position to remain calm and tackle the resolution and support phases of the PE. However, he did not let either the client or the nurse avoid the consequences of the situation. By getting the client to discuss the event with the nurse at a later date he ensured that the client faced up to the realities of her actions, and the nurse was able to debrief about her own performance, while hopefully re-establishing a working relationship with the client.

Conclusion

For obvious reasons confrontational PEs offer serious threat of personal harm to nurses. However, there are danger signals which, if spotted in time, can be used to defuse a situation before it gets out of hand. Those signals may be environmental, sociological, biological, psychological or emotional. They may appear in the client, or manifest themselves in the nurse. Either way, they are observations which must not be ignored, and need to be acted upon.

Responses need to be immediate, must protect those involved, be simple and unambiguous and non-threatening. They must be based upon a quick assessment of the situation, informing a simple game plan which involves no physical contact and no heroics.

Nurses need confidence in themselves to be able to deal effectively with an aggressive PE. This confidence often occurs because the nurse does not see the threat of violence as being personal to them, which in turn increases their potential to behave competently. The confidence for such self-efficacy often results from having a game plan, or plan of action, i.e. knowing what it is that you are going to do, and what effect it is going to have.

References

Bandura, A. (1982). Self-efficacy mechanisms in human agency. *American Psychologist*, **37**:122–47.

Cahill, C. D., Stuart, G. W., Laraira, M. T. and Arana, G. W. (1991). Inpatient management of violent behaviour: nursing prevention and intervention. *Issues in Mental Health Nursing*, **12**:239–52.

Department of Health Advisory Committee (1988). *Report: Violence to Staff*. HMSO, London.

Gluck, M. (1981). Learning a therapeutic verbal response to anger. *Journal of Psychosocial Nursing and Mental Health Services*, **19**(3):9–12.

Johnston, J. B. (1987). Violence in the emergency department. *Emergency Nursing Reports*, **1**(12):1–7.

Jones, D. and Littler, A. (1992). *Management of Violent or Potentially Violent Persons*, 2nd edn. South Glamorgan Health Authority, Cardiff.

Neades, B. L. (1994). How to handle aggression. *Emergency Nursing Reports*, **2**(2):21–4.

Podrasky, D. and Sexton, D. (1988). Nurses' reaction to difficult patients. *Image*, **20**:16–21.

Smith, M. E. and Hart, G. (1994). Nurses' responses to patient anger: from disconnecting to connecting. *Journal of Advanced Nursing*, **20**:643–51.

Turnbull, M. E., Aitken, I., Black, L. and Patterson, B. (1990). Turn it around: short term management of aggression and anger. *Journal of Psychosocial Nursing and Mental Health Services*, **28**:7–11.

Suggested reading

Cahill, C. D., Stuart, G. W., Laraira, M. T. and Arana, G. W. (1991). Inpatient management of violent behaviours: nursing prevention and intervention isuues. *Issues in Mental Health Nursing*,

12:239–52. (The authors explore a variety of preventative and predictive techniques, though the paper does cover the intervention of aggressive PEs in more detail.)

Finnema, E. J., Dassen, T. and Halfens, R. (1994). Aggression in psychiatry: a qualitative study focusing on the charaterization and perception of patient aggression by nurses working on psychiatric wards. *Journal of Advanced Nursing*, 19:1088–95. (This extensive paper explores both the perception of aggression and the issues surrounding the selection of appropriate intervention strategies. Causes of aggression are well covered, and interesting, especially as the nurses used in the study appear to have conflicting views with those of official mental healthcare bodies.)

Ryden, M. B. and Feldt, K. S. (1992). Goal directed care: caring for aggressive nursing home residents with dementia. *Journal of Gerontological Nursing*, 8(11):35–42. (This paper explores the difficult area of confrontational and unprovoked assault from elderly clients. In particular it highlights ways of developing game plans, both individual, and as nursing teams.)

8

Restraint and breakaway techniques

Introduction

So far the situations we have considered in previous chapters have been dealt with by the nurse using interactive techniques. Blakeslee *et al.* (1991) call this 'restraint-free care' and undoubtedly regard it as the most desirable method of dealing with any form of PE. Collins (1994) shows that most of the literature on aggression and violence deals primarily with prediction and prevention. Personal techniques and the skills required to action the AIRS framework certainly fall into that category. Authors such as Mentes and Ferrario (1989), Blomhoff *et al.* (1990) and Carnerie (1990) support such an approach and point to prevention and non-contact intervention as significant features for more effective resolution of assaultive PEs. However, there are going to be occasions when these techniques will not resolve the situation, either because the client has lost complete control of their emotional response, or because they are seriously disturbed and cannot make the appropriate intellectual and emotional connections between what is happening to them, and their perception of reality. In these circumstances, and when all else has either failed or is deemed too dangerous for either the client or the nurse, then restraint has to be considered.

Restraint is a method of physically immobilizing a client until either they regain control of their emotional responses, or further professional support arrives to help deal more effectively with the PE. Its use has to be carefully monitored and evaluated, for it would be easy to suggest that every time a nurse made physical contact with a client, this could be called restraint, which in turn, and in some convoluted way, justified this form of intervention. The fact is that simply grabbing hold of a client, because the nurse wants to stop him/her from doing something which the nurse sees as inappropriate or harmful, might be considered an assault rather than restraint (Miller and Maier 1987). Perhaps more significantly by simply grabbing hold of a client, without giving thought to the methods used, both the client and the nurse may be at risk of further harm, either to each other in the case of an assaultive PE, or others in situations where third parties are involved. And why, you might ask, would such an intervention be used by a nurse? The spontaneous grabbing of a client by a nurse is often the result of a loss of control by that nurse, not necessarily warranted by the client's behaviour, and possibly avoidable with forethought and self-awareness.

The nurse's self-efficacy plays a considerable part here (Collins 1994). If the nurse is confident, has thought through the interaction and planned what his/her approach is going to be, this will give them the confidence to act. If, however, these issues have not been considered before confronting a client, the nurse is more likely to feel threatened and unsupported. The resultant reduction in personal confidence this brings about may well prompt the nurse to act out of desperation and grab hold of the client, rather than through professionalism and be able to talk it out (Thackery 1987). Other factors which might motivate such unprofessional behaviours are well documented by Morrison (1990) and include such things as loss of face, embarrassment and the tradition of toughness wrongly attributed to mental health nurses.

Restraint and AIRS

Restraint, within the professional context of nursing, is not just making physical contact with a client, it is a planned, controlled and rational part of the client's care (Morning 1994). Planned, because the nursing team will have organized themselves so that when restraint is called for each individual knows their role and responsibilities. Controlled, because the procedures and training for undertaking restraint in a safe and competent way will have been dealt with before its use, and rational, because circumstances will dictate the use of restraint, either because all else has failed and it is a clinical imperative that action be taken, or because the extremes of danger dictate its use.

When the possibility of restraint becomes part of a client's care package, in other words when the nursing care plan identifies circumstances in which it is to be used, the AIRS process has already begun. The four components of the framework correlate with similar components in the restraint process.

1. **Assessment** This is the identified need for restraint, either as part of an on-going programme of intervention, or as a response to a current situation.
2. **Intervention** The actual process of restraint.
3. **Resolution** Disengaging from restraint following the reduction in client aggression, and/or the client's regaining emotional control sufficiently to be able to take control of their own actions without putting themselves or others at risk.
4. **Support** Staying with the client following the PE to discuss both the incident and the restraint. Team, or individual nurse debriefing to discuss the implications and effects of the event. This is also the time to evaluate the effectiveness of the intervention and the performance of those involved.

Methods of restraint

It is beyond the scope of this text to enter into the various forms of restraint that are available. These issues are dealt with far more effectively by practical workshops designed to teach nurses hands-on skills and provide the confidence to be able to use these skills. However, there are certain key issues which can be covered here and which might give guidance to nurses who have not had the opportunity to attend preparatory workshops, but who are nonetheless called upon to use restraint.

The need for restraint must always be documented in the client's care plan, and if it has had to be used without prior assessment recognizing its need, the care plans will need to be modified accordingly. Restraint should be avoided if the nurse is unsupported, or if colleagues are unable to provide back-up because of other commitments. The nurse initiating restraint once an assaultive PE has begun needs to know that s/he can summon support immediately. Unlike other PEs it is unlikely that team members can be gathered to effect total restraint either as the PE begins, or at the flashpoint. Therefore the nurse's awareness of the position of his/her colleagues as an assault becomes more likely is of paramount importance.

As a rule restraint ought not be undertaken by less than two nurses, and for safety's sake, preferably more. However, like all rules this one does not take account of the fact that a great many assaultive PEs take place between one client and one nurse. If the nurse really has no option left but to use restraint in a one-to-one PE then the following is just as applicable to them as it is to a well-organized nursing team.

- The nurse must get as close to the client as possible, in other words wrapping him/herself around the client in a bear hug with the client's arm pinned to his/her side. The nurse should place their head on the client's shoulder, or into their chest to avoid being butted, and keep their legs closed. Apart from reducing the possibility of being struck this position also gives the nurse time to think about what to do next.
- Call for assistance, if it has not already arrived. Do not let other clients come to your aid, but ask them to get other nurses.
- Keep talking to the client in as reassuring and calm a voice as can be managed.
- Do not let go of the client until absolutely sure that the flashpoint has passed.

When there is more than one nurse involved in the restraint, and some authors believe that three nurses are required for this procedure, they should function as a co-ordinated team. One nurse should assume the role of leader and all decisions about the length of restraint, and its discontinuation, must be made by the team leader. Where possible the client should be gently lowered to the floor during the restraint process because it is easier to pinion arms and legs against the floor, and less likely that anyone will get hurt. Team principles will include:

- Legs and arms being held at the joints to reduce the risk of fracture and inhibit client movement. Remember, the main object is to immobilize the client, not allow just enough movement so that s/he can break their own limbs.
- A nurse should lie across the client's body, effectively pinning the waist and abdomen.
- In extreme cases clients will react very violently to such restraint. Butting with the head has already been mentioned, but clients may try to bite, and the head ought to be held back in such cases.
- As with the single nurse example above, the client should only be released from such restraint when the team leader is convinced that it is safe to do so, i.e. once the flashpoint has passed. The leader will decide whether this is done by each nurse releasing one after the other, thus testing the level of control the client has, or whether all the team release in one co-ordinated movement.

Some consideration should be given to the environment when such interventions are undertaken. If other clients, visitors, patients or residents are witness to the event, it may be just as distressing for them as for those actively involved. This has implications both for support activities, but also for the assaultive client. Where possible the client should be allowed the opportunity for privacy, and this might mean removing him/her to a quieter area, or one which allows the client to work through personal feelings without upsetting others.

Finally, once the process of disengagement is complete, and the client is no longer restrained, a nurse must remain in contact with the client so that the resolution phase can be reinforced and the support necessary to effect some therapeutic rewards for the restraint be implemented. There is no way of knowing how long this phase will take. Nurses will need to work in collaboration to ensure that a rota is maintained, thus highlighting the importance given to ensuring that the client regains control and dignity, and the reasons for the assault are dealt with, rather than being ignored. However, the PE will in effect be over once the disengagement is complete.

Clients who have been restrained have more than the cause of their assault, and its impact upon the care, to deal with.

Being held forcibly against your wishes is far more dehumanizing than other, less extreme, interventions. The nurse must recognize this before beginning the long period of reconciliation that will ensue.

Consider the following example of an assaultive PE where restraint had to be used.

William was standing in his room, shouting at no-one in particular, that they could come as soon as they liked, but they would never get him to submit. This had been going on all morning, and despite several attempts at trying to get him to discuss what it was he was shouting about, William had refused. He stayed quiet for about ten minutes, and then started shouting again. He refused to come out of his room, and just appeared to be moving in a cycle of anger, and relative calm.

The nurses had decided not to antagonize him by asking questions, or trying to get him to do things he did not wish to do. He was not disturbing anyone else and his pattern of behaviour, though noisy, was one that they had seen him use before to resolve the feelings he had about certain members of his family. One nurse had spoken to William during a quite period to tell him that she, or one of her colleagues, would be close at hand should he want to talk to them. He didn't. She had discussed this approach with her team and they had agreed to keep a discreet eye on William while he was upset, to make themselves available if he needed them, but otherwise to keep a low profile unless there was a change in his behaviour which might warrant a more positive intervention.

As the morning progressed William did not settle. He became louder and the periods of time between his apparent calm got less and less. The team discussed the options open to them and agreed that someone was going to have to spend some time with William, whether he liked it or not. They also recognized that this form of confrontation, no matter how sensitively it was undertaken, might also provoke an aggressive response from William. They therefore planned for possible restraint. The team leader was appointed and responsibilities for restraint points identified. When the next calm period arrived the nurse entered William's room to talk to him, while the other two nurses waited out of sight outside.

At first things went well and it seemed as if restraint would not be necessary. William agreed to talk about what he was feeling, and even went as far as saying that he thought he was being a little unreasonable and apologized for the noise he had been making. However, he also said that it was, of course, not his fault. The nurse asked him what he meant and he began to shout that she ought to know, because she was responsible for his being there in the first place. The nurse tried to get some clarity back into the conversation but William was becoming agitated by her presence

Before she knew what had happened William sprang at her and made an attempt to strike her with his fist. The nurse responded by ducking the punch and stepping inside his reach, at the same time grabbing hold of both his arms so that he could not swing them. She shouted to her colleagues who immediately ran into the room. One held William from behind, the other held his lower limbs and feet together. The three of them held William in such a way as he could not move, but he was struggling ferociously, so the leader co-ordinated lowering him to the floor, where they were able to restrain him more effectively, with less likelihood of anyone being hurt.

All the time this was taking place the nurse was taking to William in as calm a voice as possible. No-one else spoke so that William was able to concentrate on what was being said to him. The nurse told him that he was all right, and that they were only holding him so that he did not hurt anyone, including himself. She kept talking, even when William tried to shout her down. She kept repeating that he was safe, and would come to no harm. He asked angry questions about why he needed to be held as he was, and the nurse answered his questions directly, and truthfully. She also said that she was frightened by his anger, and frightened too that he might hurt himself or others. He said he did not want to hurt anyone, and apologized for trying to hit her. She, as the leader of the team, had to decide when, and how to release William. She felt that the flashpoint had gone, and decided to withdraw slowly. First the nurse lying across William's waist let go and knelt back out of the way; then the nurse restraining the legs and finally herself. Once she was satisfied that William was not going to strike out again, the first nurse stood up and left the room, shortly afterwards the second one did too. All the time the leader was signalling this to take place she was talking quietly to William, trying to get him to discuss what was going on.

The whole activity took about 15 minutes from the time that she had first been attacked to the moment when the second nurse left the room. Though they stood outside, as agreed beforehand, for several minutes it was obvious that William had settled considerably and was at last discussing the event quietly. They left the nurse to carry on, but remained alert to any call for help that she might make, when the whole procedure would be repeated if necessary.

The two nurses took it in turn to relieve the lead nurse and, as they did, so the remaining pair of nurses acted as a support for each other. They considered their actions, and the outcome of their intervention, recorded the event in William's care documents, and amended his care plan to take into consideration feelings they had about their approach. They also discussed this in depth with William so that he could contribute to the support and after-care of the PE.

From this example it can be seen that planning to restrain does not necessarily mean that restraint will take place. However, having the back-up for restraint does give the nurse the confidence, or self-efficacy, to explore more rigorously, some of the alternatives. In this case it did not work, but the professional way in which the restraint was undertaken enabled a positive outcome to the PE.

AIRS was used in the assessment of William's behaviour, and his potential for aggression; in the development of a plan for intervention which was put into operation the moment it was needed. The resolution to the PE came while William was being restrained, and he was not released until the nurse was sure that it had occurred. Finally, support for both the team members and William himself was offered and given in a variety of ways.

Of course this example of restraint benefitted from having the right amount of staff, with the right amount of time, to carry out the procedure correctly. For many nurses this may not be the case. They may be under-resourced, under-staffed, have other clients demanding their attention or be unprepared because of a lack of information about the potentially assaultive client. A client being seen for the first time, one being admitted, someone that the nurse is unfamiliar with, or someone to whom something extraordinary has happened, may all fall into this category. The nurse has to recognize that such events may occur and plan for them, long before making client contact.

Nurses must be aware of the resources available to them, must plan effective restraint strategies, and develop a practice of lead roles that can be utilized in any situation. Being flexible to the needs of the PE as well as those of the client is the key to success here. It is also important to recognize that once restraint has been used nurses are going to be committed to that role for some time, at least until resolution of the PE, and possibly longer if the client is very disturbed. All these issues have to be considered when contemplating restraint, and all must be incorporated into the working procedure that ensues.

Breakaway techniques

Restraint may be one alternative open to a nurse being assaulted, but what if the client is extremely violent in the attack, is much bigger than the nurse, or there is no possibility of any immediate support? What if holding on to the client in one-to-one restraint is totally inappropriate? Some other form of safety mechanism must be available to the nurse.

During recent years techniques have been developed which are designed to get nurses out of difficult and potentially dangerous situations quickly and at no risk to themselves. Most of these techniques are hold-breaking, or distractive manoeuvres, and nearly all demand that once they have been used the nurse gets away from the client as quickly as possible to summon support. Many of these techniques are painful to the client, as in the case of the nurse stamping on the toes of a client who has grabbed her from behind, and as such they appear to contradict the professional code of conduct which insists that nurses shall not harm their clients in any way. However, what we are talking about here is not sustained pain for the sake of it, but a short, sharp shock to get the nurse free from a potentially life-threatening PE. As a result the nurse will be in a better position to help the client, than if s/he is incapacitated or in need of medical help.

These techniques, generally known as breakaway techniques, are not all painful to the client. For example, if a client becomes angry and grabs hold of the nurse's clothing, the natural tendency is to try to break free. The result however, will probably be torn clothing. It is much better to move towards the force of the pull so that the client cannot do any damage. The same applies to hair pulling. Many elderly clients use this behaviour to protect themselves against what they see as a serious threat to them, i.e. the nurse trying to help. They grab hold of the person's hair, shouting for someone to come to their assistance, while the nurse does their best to extricate themselves from this apparently fragile old lady with the vice-like grip of a Japanese sumo wrestler. Moving away from the grip is extremely painful, and cutting the hair with a pair of scissors is the stuff of nightmares. The nurse must lean forward into the force of the pulling until the client is not able to exert any pull at all. Obviously the nurse must also be careful not to attract other forms of retribution while being so close!

As with restraint, this text cannot teach breakaway techniques. They have to be practised under the supervision of experts. What this text can do is urge the reader to seek out those experts. Learning a few simple activities, such as rubbing hard at the base of the client's sternum as he tries to strangle you, just long enough for you to get away, or breaking the bear-hug from the rear by forcing the client's little fingers apart, may mean the difference between being able to resolve an assaultive PE or being seriously injured.

Conclusion

This, and the previous two chapters, have considered a variety of aggressive and violent PEs. The emphasis has been placed firmly upon the prediction of such events by a careful monitoring of the client's behaviour, by an understanding of the nurse's impact upon that behaviour, and on an understanding of human behaviour generally. What this chapter has done is explore situations where talking alone will not bring the PE to a successful conclusion.

The use of restraint must be seen as a last resort, but as with every other technique or procedure it must be planned, implemented, resolved and supported. In many ways it is because the nurse, or a nursing team, have to use restraint which makes the method of its application more important. Restraining someone is not only undignified for all concerned, it can be dangerous if not carried out properly, therefore being responsible in planning for its use is as important as the enlightenment needed to implement it properly.

Post-assaultive PE support is likely to be more time-consuming and involved if restraint has been used. This needs to be recognized when restraint is being discussed or planned, for cutting corners in care by denying clients the right amount of time for support following such events is only likely to increase the possibility of their happening again.

Finally, it cannot be stressed enough at this point that nurses who have been assaulted, or attacked, or just threatened with violence, need time to recover afterwards, and the support of their colleagues to do so.

References

Blakeslee, J. A., Goldman, B. D., Popougenis, D. and Torell, C. A. (1991). Making the transition to restraint-free care. *Journal of Gerontological Nursing*, 17(2):4–8.

Blomhoff, S., Seim, S. and Friis, S. (1990). Can prediction of violence among psychiatric in-patients be improved? *Hospital and Community Psychiatry*, 41(7):771–5.

Carnerie, F. (1990). Violence against nurses: an ounce of prevention is worth a pound of cure. *The Registered Nurse*, 2(1):42–3.

Collins, J. (1994). Nurses' attitudes towards aggressive behaviour following attendance at 'The Prevention and Management of Aggressive Behaviour Programme'. *Journal of Advanced Nursing*, 20:117–31.

Mentes, J. C. and Ferrario, J. (1989). Calming aggressive reactions: a preventative program. *Journal of Gerontological Nursing*, 15(2):22–7.

Miller, R. D. and Maier, G. J. (1987). Factors affecting the decision to prosecute mental patients for criminal behaviour. *Hospital and Community Psychiatry*, 38:50–4.

Morning, D. (1994). Coping with violence: workshops for CPNs. *Nursing Standard*, 8(23):30–3.

Morrison, E. F. (1990). The tradition of toughness: a study of non-professional nursing care in psychiatric settings. *Image: Journal of Nursing Scholarship*, 22(1):32–8.

Thackery, M. (1987). Clinician confidence in coping with patient aggression: assessment and enhancement. *Professional Psychology: Research and Practice*, 18:57–60.

Suggested reading

Outlaw, F. W. and Lowery, B. J. (1994). An attributional study of seclusion and restraint of psychiatric patients. *Archives of Psychiatric Nursing*, 8(2):69–77. (The main reason for selecting this paper is its discussion on the different views about restraint held by clients, and the nurses who restrained them. Clients identify situational causes, i.e. because I hit him, whereas the nurses identify dispositional ones, i.e. he was a danger to himself or others.)

Snyder, J. A. (1993). Documentation of nursing care for patients who have been restrained. *Journal of Emergency Nursing*, 19(5):461–4. (The article considers a system for recording the restraint process. It highlights the problems associated with post-event recording, but shows that by using a well-managed system decisions can be made about resourcing restraint activities.)

Splawn, G. (1991). Restraining potentially violent patients. *Journal of Emergency Nursing*, 17(5):316–17. (The article deals with the author's views on safe restraint, guidelines for the care of restrained clients, and an exercise to help staff understand what it is like to be restrained.)

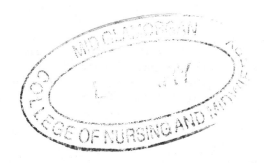

9

Care confrontations

Introduction

In the previous three chapters we have considered problems
associated with aggression and violence, and their impact upon
possible psychiatric emergencies (PEs). We have also looked at
the way AIRS (Assessment, Intervention, Resolution and
Support) can be used, firstly to detect the potential for such
PEs, but also as a framework for managing them effectively
once they occur. In this chapter we will explore some of the
circumstances within a clinical environment which might
potentiate PEs, and in particular address issues which are
directly related to the care process.

There is a twofold purpose for such an approach. Firstly, it
provides the opportunity to explore certain nursing activities
which, though perhaps routine for the most part, may provoke
extreme reactions from some clients, and secondly, to look at
the effects of more ill-conceived nursing actions. By comparing
the two it may be possible to develop guidelines for good
practice when dealing with care management issues.

Management of care issues

If a client refuses to take prescribed medication, or wishes to
leave the hospital precinct while on a restriction order, it is
invariably the nurse's responsibility to deal with these events. In
certain situations the nurse has enough leeway to be able to
compromise and as a result no confrontation occurs. However,

in other situations there may not be that room for compromise. In that event the nurse will have to work extremely hard to ensure that the priorities of a client's care are adhered to while attempting to avoid direct confrontation. Managing care is not just a question of ensuring that a client's care plan is followed, or that it is reviewed on time and appropriate modifications made. It is also about providing a climate in which these activities can take place effectively. Sometimes referred to as the therapeutic milieu, this climate involves ensuring that a client is in the right place at the right time, getting the right care, in the right way. How it is produced will depend entirely upon the clients and nurses involved, and upon the procedures and practices of the organization, but, if issues of managing care are not addressed in the same strategic way that care plan issues are, then they are just as likely to produce PEs.

Care management, at a clinical level, represents those activities that a nurse will be involved in which surround the central core of the care plan. They may, or may not, be identified implicitly on a care plan, and they may arise as a direct result of prescribed care decisions. Unless specifically thought through beforehand, their resolution will require quick thinking by the nurse, and can easily result in some form of client/nurse confrontation if the thinking is unsound, or the decision appears unfair.

Finnema *et al.* (1994) found that many nurses working on psychiatric wards experienced aggression and violence in ways dissimilar to that of people who were less likely to be involved in it. In particular they found that nurses viewed aggression as being situational, or responsive, rather than characteristic of the client behaviour. In other words, while there is evidence to show that some clients are habitually aggressive (Lanza 1983, Convit 1990) nurses feel that it is circumstances that produce aggression, and subsequent PEs, not necessarily the client. It would therefore seem sensible to develop and maintain care plan and care management continuity.

Before such a situation exists it has to be recognized that care will almost definitely produce conflicts of interest between nurses, who represent the care group, and clients, who represent the group for whom care is intended. The conflict may arise as a consequence of the nurse's not listening to the client, thus failing to recognize essential needs, or it may arise as a direct result of the care being too challenging for the client to cope with. The skill of good care management is being able to recognize where these discrepancies may occur and dealing with them before a PE takes place.

Generally speaking it is possible to monitor the effects of care planning on a client by considering the impact that care will have. The impact may be a set of events, such as wanting to leave contrary to professional advice, or a reaction such as a violent response after being refused immediate access to case documents. The impact represents care management, and as such is a continuum of the care process. Decisions made about the care plan may therefore have both a direct and indirect effect upon the whole of the care process, with consequences represented as care management issues.

Management of care and AIRS

Once the nurse recognizes that caring can become something of a contradiction in terms, with the client viewing care as intrusive and threatening, while the nurses forge on regardless with the absolute conviction that what they are doing is in the client's best interest, then positive steps can be taken to promote the therapeutic milieu (Tmobranski 1994). The object is to produce a situation in which clients and nurses can work in collaboration, thus reducing the tension of conflict and confrontation. It would, of course, be foolish to suggest that all tension and confrontation can be removed from a professional relationship, or indeed to deny that confrontation is a therapeutic tool within certain clinical strategies. However, what we are considering here is the environment in which these strategies, and other less challenging ones, may be implemented. It may be an in-patient facility, or a community one. Nurses may have regular contact with the client 24 hours a day, or once a fortnight, but the issues remain the same.

AIRS, as we have seen in Chapters 5–7, may be used to determine both the nature of a client's response to the care programme, as well as a method for planning what to do once the response has generated some form of PE. In planning to reduce the potential for a PE within care management the same principles apply.

- **Assessment** – involves establishing the consequences of care planning decisions. The nurse uses his/her knowledge of human behaviour as a baseline, but also past experience of clinical decision-making. All actions will have reactions, and the nurse will know that if a patient is going to be asked difficult and potentially painful questions about their problems, they may respond aggressively. Assessing the client's potential for violence has to be carried out by placing it against the impact that the care process may have upon him/her.
- **Intervention** – involves taking the assessment information and planning a suitably responsive strategy for counteracting any potentially volatile aspects of it. Of course, it may be necessary for the client to experience the depths of their own feelings, but this has to be done in such a way as to avoid coming to any physical harm. The intervention will need to involve a default component, which covers the eventuality that the client may over-respond to the care, or indeed, respond differently than expected. This default will include the game plan for dealing with the PE if it occurs.
- **Resolution** – as always is the reduction of the emotional energy within a PE to a level which enables either the client to resume control over their own actions or the nurse or nursing team to maintain safe status until such time as the client is in a position to do so. In situations which involve conflict over care decisions such as leave, medication or freedom of movement, it is likely that one flashpoint may lead to another while an eventual agreement is sought. Resolution at such times may therefore be rather transitory.
- **Support** – for the nurses involved has to begin before the PE does, during it and afterwards. For the client it begins once the flashpoint has been reached and carries on through resolution of the PE and into the more long-term crisis intervention that might follow. The support would not be discontinued till it was felt that all those receiving it no longer required it, or, in the case of extreme response to the PE, had been referred to more long term supportive agencies, i.e.

nurse support group or counselling service for the nurse, therapeutic counselling or care revision for the client.

There are three main considerations here. When AIRS is used effectively it is because

1. Baseline behaviours and therapeutic responses have been considered in detail by the nursing team, in conjunction with medical and non-medical colleagues of the multi-disciplinary team.
2. Care plan development, that part of the care process which is closest to the client, has been carried out in a collaborative spirit, with both the client and the nurse having real input.
3. Genuine equality is experienced by the client and the nurse. This may be hard to achieve, especially if the nurse always appears to make all the decisions, but can be done if the nurse allows the client full access to the decision-making process.

Confrontation events

While it would not be possible to list all the confrontational situations which might lead to a violent or aggressive PE, there are certain situations which can be identified as being more difficult than others. The following is not intended to be a definitive list, merely an indication of the sort of circumstances that may cause problems within care management. It does not deal with issues related to diagnosis and/or mental status which are dealt with in the next chapter.

- **Any situation where confrontation is inevitable**. This is likely to be related to prescribed care, medications, treatments, investigations, that the client does not want, will not have, and refuses to discuss. Longo (1993) sees this as clients withdrawing from treatment and describes it as a quality of life issue. Certainly, unless clients can see the rightness of the nurse's course of action there is always the potential for a PE.
- **Leaving against professional advice**. In some situations the client is at liberty to make this decision, but in others,

either because some form of lawful restriction order exists and the nurse has to abide by it, or because the nurse is genuinely concerned about the safety or welfare of the client, the client may not have the same degree of responsibility (Weissburg *et al.* 1986, Green 1988). The nurse may have no choice here and the presence of a predetermined strategy for dealing with this event may provide enough support to deflect the possible PE.

- **Non-co-operation with routines and in-house practices**. At first sight this might seem a strange thing to suggest, but it does not relate so much to client–staff confrontation but to client-client confrontation. This is particularly the case in hostels or small centres where each client is expected to conform to certain sociological norms. These may have been laid down by the organization, though the more effective ones are those agreed among the residents or clients themselves. If one client appears to flout the rules, or does not appear to be contributing to the general good in the same way that the other group members are, this is grounds for injustice. Clients are just as likely to respond to injustice from other clients, as they are from nurses. The example in Chapter 7, with the loud radio, could easily have been prompted by another client rather than the nurse. Wanting to watch television late at night, demanding access to foodstuffs, night drinks or alcohol, are all likely to generate conflict with staff members, but may also irritate other clients.

- **Client to client conflict generally**. This is often caused because one client's mental disturbance causes distress, annoyance or frustration to others. The nurse has to recognize the irritation being generated, or the client may be at risk of being attacked by another client. Such behaviours are often seen in areas for the elderly mentally ill, or admission areas where some clients are considerably unwell, and others are not.

- **Care plan conflicts**. If the care plan has been developed without the client's knowledge or consent confrontation becomes a definite possibility. This issue has already been discussed above but the sort of problems that it can generate range from clients being expected to participate in care activities which they do not like, feel threatened by or are unexplained, to those which demand their co-operation at times when they are least likely to be able to take part, during visiting hours for example.

- **Where certain predetermined factors inhibit a client from responding appropriately**. This relates more directly to the reactionary nature of a client's condition, such as acting out behaviour in adolescents (Muscari 1992), or difficulties associated with eating disorders (Love and Seaton 1991). Although this and other diagnostic issues are dealt with in Chapter 10, nurses need to be aware that each individual condition does have its own special areas of concern, and each has to be considered against the client behaviour, the care process and nature of the therapeutic milieu.

- **Response to dignity, freedom and privacy issues** (Muscari 1992). Certainly every nurse is aware of the basics of privacy, allowing clients to undertake very personal human actions, such as bathing or going to the toilet, in a dignified way. But what of the situation where there is no lock on the bathroom door for fear of clients locking themselves in and drowning in the bath? What of the situation where clients are given plastic cutlery in case they cut themselves or others? What of situations where a client is not allowed to close the door to his/her room, or is not allowed to get dressed during the day but has to walk about in a dressing gown? Are these situations, and many others besides, deemed necessary in some centres for safety purposes, dignified? Do they restrict privacy for a purpose, and can the purpose be defended? Either way, they represent serious implications for the development of PEs and nurses must be aware that along the care continuum the implications may sometimes warrant a rethink of the care process.

Effects upon the client

For the nurse to be able to detect the potential for a PE s/he must be able to observe the changes in client behaviour consistent with the event. This baseline is an essential ingredient in predicting such events. Consider the following example.

James had asked for a meeting with his primary nurse just after breakfast. It had been agreed that they would meet later in the morning, though no specific time had been mentioned. As the morning progressed it became obvious that James was becoming increasingly agitated. He was pacing the ward incessantly, would not talk to anyone, and kept asking where Peter, the nurse, had got to. Other members of staff who tried to talk to him were cut short by James who simply walked away and left them.

Peter was working with two other clients, but his colleagues informed him of James' condition. He made a point of going to talk to James at about 11.15 a.m., but only to tell James that he would have to wait a little longer, and that perhaps they could meet before lunch. James was unhappy about this, and made Peter promise that he would see him.

When lunchtime came Peter still had not had the opportunity to see James, who by now was causing concern, not just to the other nurses with whom he would not make contact, but to other clients who were becoming irritated by his constant pacing. Peter asked one of his colleagues to tell James he would be about five minutes. He went to make himself a cup of coffee, having just had a difficult session with another client. He sat down to write up his notes and was interrupted twice by telephone enquiries. Half an hour later he went in search of James, but could not find him. He asked the other nurses where he was and they eventually found him walking in the grounds.

Peter met him at the door, apologizing for being so late and explaining what had transpired. James hit him very hard in the face with a fist-sized stone he had picked up in the gardens.

The issue here is not about whether or not Peter or any of the nurses were at fault, or even if James was pushed into taking the action he did. The question is about the baseline behaviour, James's previous history and the care management sequence. The nurses were aware that James was becoming more and more distressed, and though they made an effort to connect with him, they saw it as Peter's responsibility to help James. Peter had other things to do, other clients to see, and a busy care diary to work with. James's request to see him was on top of the other things he had planned and did not warrant becoming a priority at the time the meeting was arranged. The morning's events led to the PE, and to an extent Peter and his colleagues were to blame.

Keeping people waiting causes no end of stress, but it is not so much the wait as not knowing when it is going to end which generates the stress. For a person experiencing distressing and frightening feelings, who has difficulty controlling their emotions, who trusts another sufficiently that they will not speak with others, such a wait becomes almost impossible to bear. Peter, of course, could not have known this when he initially spoke to James, but he should have been more honest about the amount of time he was going to be, he could have been more specific about the meeting time itself, and he should not have disappointed James by apparently meeting him, only to tell him that their meeting would be later than intended.

The other nurses should have realized that James was reaching flashpoint, should have kept Peter better informed and should not have agreed to act as a 'go-between' for Peter. They may have been able to help with the work that Peter was already involved in, but even if not, should have kept a better eye on James, and tried to support him more constructively than they did.

> As soon as James hit Peter with the stone he fell to the floor. Other nurses ran to his aid and a female client started to scream. The nurses did not try to talk to James, but grabbed him, lowered him to the floor and restrained him using rehearsed control techniques. Peter, bleeding badly from the mouth, was unable to talk properly and was led away. James, more angry than ever now, was shouting at the top of his voice. Different combinations of team members spent nearly two and a half hours with him during the afternoon, and again during the evening trying to help him. He had wanted clarification about his medication, which Peter could have given in considerably less time, and far more effectively.
>
> Peter was off sick for three weeks; James was identified as a potentially dangerous client and had his medication increased.

Keeping clients waiting is just one of a long list of personal difficulties that might arise in a busy clinical environment, but the message here is about recognition of client behaviour, staff honesty and time-keeping. The client kept waiting is the client who feels that he or she is not important enough to be seen on time, whose problems are not seen as important or which simply do not warrant the same attention as others. This frustrating and humiliating response may easily lead to aggression and the flashpoint of a violent PE. The client may see the nurse as the perpetrator of aggression, shouting the client down or denying them the same rights as other clients.

There are other such actions which fall into this category, not necessarily prompted by nurses, but certainly exacerbated by events which take place within the management of care.

- failing to keep appointments;
- failing to comply with care plan statements, and expecting the client to go along with you;
- not doing what you said you would do;
- reducing the client's involvement so that they become disempowered;
- changing plans without letting the client know;
- asking clients to do things of which they do not think they are capable;
- asking the client to do things which they find frightening; this may be part of a perfectly legitimate therapy programme, for example, desensitization, but it needs careful handling and considerable client support;
- putting clients under pressure to comply with care programmes about which they are unhappy, or cannot understand;
- failing to communicate generally about care, therapy or treatment issues;
- making clients feel embarrassed, especially in relation to issues connected with their sexuality, personal background, drinking or lifestyle problems (McMahon and Jones 1992);
- making clients feel ashamed, in relation to sexuality, abuse or personal status (Smith 1992);
- neglecting the impact of psychological problems upon the client's ability to control, or correctly perceive the necessity to control, their emotions. This is particularly relevant to those who are severely disturbed, or some elderly mentally ill clients with serious short term memory difficulties (Rossby *et al.* 1992);
- response to physical pain (May 1991);
- response to psychological pain (Cahill *et al.* 1991);
- response to change (Norman and Parker 1990).

Responding to the client's needs

Even the best planned strategies can go wrong. Sometimes the PE is suspected, but its flashpoint is so rapid that all the nurse can do is respond as effectively as possible, while trying to stick to a previously agreed game plan. However, if the nurse has some understanding of what it is the client is seeking from such behaviour it may be possible to manipulate the care environment to such a degree that this can be achieved. Even if this is not possible the recognition by the nurse that the client has a definite reason for their behaviour, and that the nurse has some understanding of that reason, may be enough at least to begin the process of diffusing the PE.

The following example occurred after Grace, an elderly lady with severe memory problems, had not been visited by the psychiatric nurse working in the community, in this case a qualified community psychiatric nurse (CPN), for several days. Grace lived with her daughter and while there was some tension in the house, generally speaking they got on quite well. There had been several incidents of verbal abuse in the past months as Grace's condition had began to deteriorate and the daughter had found it increasingly difficult to keep Grace occupied, or cheerful.

The visit followed the usual pattern. Grace, the daughter and the CPN sat in the lounge and discussed what had happened since the last visit. It was obvious that Grace could not remember who the CPN was and some time was spent trying to help her, but with no success. In fact Grace was obviously irritated by the suggestion that she might be ill and therefore need the attention of a nurse. She asked the CPN to leave and when she did not do so immediately became abusive both towards the nurse and the daughter. Eventually they left Grace in the lounge and moved into the kitchen. They discussed the problems that had arisen and the daughter assured the CPN that she was quite able to cope at the moment, and that her mother would soon settle down if the nurse were to leave.

They agreed the time and date of the next visit.

However, before leaving the CPN asked the daughter what provisions she had made to defend herself against any possible violence from Grace. At first the daughter was a little taken aback by this but soon realized the necessity of such a plan. For about five minutes the CPN outlined a few key points that she thought might help the daughter and then the two of them walked through the house towards the front door. As they did so Grace came out of the lounge and met them in the hall. She had no recollection of who either of them were and was obviously taken aback at seeing two people in what she had assumed was an empty house.

Screaming in fright she grabbed hold of her daughter's hair and pulled her violently towards her. At first the daughter tried to pull away, but this only made Grace more determined to hang on. She stopped screaming as she concentrated on trying to pull the hair from her daughter's head. She started to call her daughter Margaret, not her name, and accused her of coming into her house to steal her money.

The CPN was pushed away from the two of them by the initial attack and was unable to get around the daughter to intervene for quite some time. Her intention was to try to get between the two of them, but she soon realized that this would make matters worse. Instead she gently pushed the two of them into the lounge where she knew a sofa was placed in the far side of the room. As she did so she tried to keep the daughter as close to Grace as possible so that there was less chance of the hair-pulling hurting the daughter. She also realized that Grace was frightened, and had been startled, and was now determined to defend herself. The daughter, in some pain but relieved by the CPN's action, asked what to do, while allowing herself to be moved into the lounge.

The CPN reminded her of the conversation they had just had, and the daughter responded by telling Grace that she was hurting her, and that it was she, her daughter, of whom she had taken hold. There was no obvious response from Grace, in fact she carried on telling 'Margaret' that she would punish her. The nurse got them to the settee and very gently she and the daughter lowered themselves, and Grace, on to it. The daughter kept repeating who she was, and the nurse kept them close together. Eventually, as Grace began to question just what it was that was happening, the CPN changed the subject slightly, asking if she could help Grace and her daughter in some way. Grace was now sufficiently unsure of herself that she let go of her daughter's hair.

This is a relatively simple incident. The hair-pulling could easily have been biting, grabbing of clothes or hands and arms. The victim could have been anyone who happened to be there at the time. On this occasion the daughter was unlucky to be the closest person to Grace, and therefore the one who took the brunt of the confusion that ensued.

The PE was diffused in several ways.

1. The nurse was able to reduce the pain being inflicted by keeping Grace and the daughter very close together.

2. The CPN and the daughter had discussed 'reality speak', or repeating the truth of a situation, just minutes before the PE. Consequently the daughter had some idea of how to respond to Grace's behaviour.
3. The nurse manipulated the environment so that she could move the pair to a safer place, one which made Grace more comfortable, but also made it easier to talk to her.
4. Finally the nurse used diversionary conversation to reinforce what the daughter was saying.

Of course, after the event it was necessary to debrief the daughter, who felt both angry and frightened, and support Grace, who was not sure what had happened, but was breathless and shaking.

In this case the nurse knew that what Grace was seeking was the reassurance that she was safe in her own home. She succeeded in creating the impression that this was the case by getting the daughter to remind her constantly who she was and, when the moment seemed appropriate, to change the subject slightly, and in a tone of voice which reflected familiarity. Eventually Grace felt safer and let go.

There are always going to be situations where what the client asks, and what the nurse is able to provide, conflict. Nurses cannot give drugs to those who demand them, nor can they provide alcohol, or let people die simply because they request it. What of the client who refuses to have an injection because he does not want it, yet the nurse has to give it because of legal orders? What of the client who requests to leave a clinical environment against the wishes of the care team members who are convinced that she will do serious harm to herself if she does? These, and many other situations, raise ethical as well as clinical questions about nurse decision-making, and the desire to respond to the needs and wishes of the client group.

There is no straightforward answer to any of them. Nurses need to address those questions as they occur, but also preempt them by considering the nature of the client's request, the nature of the care process and the significance of the care environment in trying to marry the two. Ultimately it may be client and nurse safety which will be the main determinant in providing the answers.

Conclusion

This chapter has tried to explore some of the issues related to the management of care. This has been placed in the context of the client, the care plan and the process of care, and has been referred to as the care environment. We have seen that in some cases manipulation of the care environment is just as crucial to the early resolution of a PE as the care plan intervention itself. Perhaps more significantly we have seen the tactics employed in earlier chapters considered in relation to this broader aspect of the caring situation. What nurses need to recognize, however, is that while it is possible to plan for certain eventualities, this does not necessarily mean that they can be averted. Similarly, some situations may occur totally unpredictably. The nurse will have to use both flexibility and ingenuity to bring about a successful resolution in both sets of circumstances. Using the needs of the client as the basis of any decision as to dealing with the PE seems to be a logical conclusion.

Finally, it is worth remembering that good verbal interaction may avert a serious PE, but there are times when it will not. On the other hand, bad interaction very rarely has the same degree of success.

References

Cahill, C. D., Stuart, G. W., Laraia, M. T. and Arana, G. W. (1991). Inpatient management of violent behaviour: nursing prevention and intervention. *Issues in Mental Health Nursing*, **12**:239–52.

Convit, A., Isay, D., Otis, D. and Volavka, J. (1990). Characteristics of repeatedly assaultive psychiatric in-patients. *Hospital and Community Psychiatry*, **41**:1112–15.

Finnema, E. J., Dassen, T. and Halfens, R. (1994). Aggression in psychiatry: a qualitative study focusing on the charaterization and perception of patient aggression by nurses working on psychiatric wards. *Journal of Advanced Nursing*, **19**:1088–95.

Green, J. H. (1988). Frequent rehospitalization and noncompliance with treatment. *Hospital and Community Psychiatry*, **39**(9):963–6.

Lanza, M. (1983). Origins of aggression. *Journal of Psychosocial Nursing and Mental Health Services*, **21**:11–16.

Longo, M. B. (1993). Facilitating acceptance of a patient's decision to stop treatment. *Clinical Nurse Specialist*, **7**(3):116–20.

Love, C. C. and Seaton, H. (1991). Eating disorders: highlights of nursing assessment and therapies. *Nursing Clinics of North America*, **26**(3):677–97.

McMahon, J. and Jones, B. T. (1992). The change process in alcoholics: client motivation and denial in the treatment of alcoholism within the context of contemporary nursing. *Journal of Advanced Nursing*, **17**:173–86.

May, C. (1991). Affective neutrality and involvement in nurse–patient relationships: perception of appropriate behaviour among nurses in acute medical and surgical wards. *Journal of Advanced Nursing*, **16**:552–8.

Meddaugh, D. I. (1992). Lack of privacy may trigger aggressive behaviors. *Provider*, **18**(7):39.

Muscari, M. E. (1992). The 'acting out' adolescent: identification and management. *Pediatric Nursing*, **18**(4):362–6.

Norman, J. and Parker, F. (1990). Psychiatric patient's views of their lives before and after moving to a hostel: a qualitative study. *Journal of Advanced Nursing*, **15**:1036–44.

Rossby, L., Beck, C. and Heacock, P. (1992). Disruptive behaviours of a cognitively impaired nursing home resident. *Archives of Psychiatric Nursing*, **6**(2): 98–107.

Smith, G. B. (1992). Nursing care challenges: homosexual psychiatric patients. *Journal of Psychosocial Nursing and Mental Health Services*, **30**(12):15–21, 37–8.

Tmobranski, P. H. (1994). Nurse-patient negotiation: assumption or reality? *Journal of Advanced Nursing*, **19**:733–7.

Weissberg, M. P., Heitner, M., Lowenstein, S. R. and Keefer, G. (1986). Patients who leave without being seen. *Annals of Emergency Medicine*, **15**:813–17.

Suggested reading

Brook, A. (1993). Emotional minefield. *Nursing Times*, **89**(3):48–9. (While this article discusses the difficult to handle client, as opposed to a psychiatric emergency, it addresses situational pressures common to both.)

Gould, J. (1994). The impact of change on violent patients. *Nursing Standard*, **8**(19):38–40. (Describes the effects of change on one ward for the long-term mentally ill, and explores the measures and techniques that were employed to reduced the levels of violence towards staff.)

Ruscitti, C. (1992). Caring for a combative patient. *Nursing*, **22**(9):50–1. (A straightforward account of the difficulties associated with difficult to handle clients, with the emphasis placed upon the care, rather than containment, issues.)

10

Emergencies associated with psychological disturbance

Introduction

Much of the literature which deals with psychiatric emergencies focuses upon the client's medical condition as a prerequisite for violent outbursts or directed aggression. It is certainly the case that many of these conditions may have extreme behavioural presentations which render the client more susceptible to a PE. However, there is some evidence to show that it is often a combination of factors, client related, situational and interactional, which cause such events (Winger *et al.* 1987, Swanson *et al.* 1990, Finnema *et al.* 1994). It is far too simplistic to suggest that, simply because a client has, say, a medical diagnosis of schizophrenia, s/he is more prone to violent outbursts than anyone else; it is also untrue. It is also equally untrue that all PEs are of a violent nature.

It is necessary to explore the concept of mental health before embarking upon the effects that the opposite might have upon the individual; therefore this chapter will begin with a comparison of the two states of mind, and then consider how mental ill health may manifest itself and raise the potential for a PE. It will also look at specific at-risk groups, some of which have already been dealt with in earlier chapters, and they will be simply revisited here.

Mental health vs mental ill health

Newnes (1993, 1994) is quite clear that mental health is characterized by a series of acts or actions which can be carried out by the individual. Conversely, when mentally unwell they are unable to undertake these activities, or at least not satisfactorily. He identifies the following – clarity of thought, kindness, calm, intimacy, enjoyment of life, the ability to work, love and co-operate with others, saying what you mean and meaning what you say. Sustaining mental health means that we are able to carry out competently those other activities we undertake, on a daily basis, which are required to bring about success, happiness and a state of well-being. These include making decisions, demonstrating self-worth, communicating effectively with others, developing and maintaining meaningful relationships, knowing our limitations, knowing when to seek help and advice, and many more. They fall into five basic categories:

1. having an appreciation of your own feelings, and accepting that you feel the way you do;
2. knowing your own failings, and those things which make you vulnerable;
3. being interested in what goes on around you and developing yourself accordingly;
4. developing meaningful relationships, and being in contact with other people;
5. knowing when you need help, and an awareness of how to go about getting it.

Mental health is a complex phenomenon and may differ from individual to individual. Jahoda (1958) was critical of simplistic definitions of mental health, stating that no single criterion could be used to measure it. If the individual is able to undertake activities associated with mental health, then facing up to change, or a challenge, or having to overcome adversity, while never easy, will not be as difficult. In a sense life is satisfying for those who are mentally well, and as such they will have less to argue or disagree about than someone who is mentally unwell. Heron (1977) identifies four dominant aspects of emotion which, in Western society, are frequently denied or repressed;

anger, grief, fear and embarrassment. All of these are difficult for anyone to deal with, but they become harder to deal with as the individual loses the ability to deal effectively with activities of daily living as expressed through mental wellness. This mental wellness can be reduced by both physical or psychological pain, rejection, self-doubt, constant criticism, a downward change in personal circumstances, loss or failure. However, in themselves, they represent a list of events or occurrences that any individual may suffer from, but some people have far greater difficulties to overcome, and it is this group for whom mental unwellness is far more significant.

Another way of viewing the health–illness phenomena is through successful problem solving (see also Chapters 1 and 3). The ability of the individual to resolve problems successfully, an adaptive response, could be seen as healthy, while the opposite, a maladaptive response, could be seen as unhealthy. Along this continuum, the less the individual is able to resolve problems the more unwell they become. As different problems arise they impact upon each other until it becomes impossible to see where one begins and any other finishes. At this point the confusing stimuli of emotion generated by the individual's lack of control over what is happening to him/her may easily predispose a PE. While it is true, therefore, that any individual may suffer a PE, those for whom successful problem-solving has become impossible or extremely difficult are more likely to experience such events. Scales which measure the amount of stress an individual is under, such as the Holmes and Rahe, Social Readjustment Rating Scale (1967) provide indicators for the level of well-being, but so too does the presence of behaviours associated with mental illness.

Psychological disturbance and the PE

For an individual to experience psychological disturbance does not necessarily mean that they are diagnosed as being mentally ill. The term applies to any situation where the individual is either unable to relate to the stimuli they are receiving, or cannot make sense of the origins of that stimuli. Such situations can happen to anyone. They can occur, for example, if someone is woken suddenly, finds themselves in unfamiliar situation, or is suffering an illness with a high temperature. Abusing alcohol or drugs may well bring about a similar response (see Chapter 11). However, it stands to reason that if an individual is having difficulties making sense of their thoughts, feelings and mental processes already, such factors put them more at risk of a PE.

Psychological disturbance can be seen as an altered state of awareness. It interferes with the individual's ability to make sense of what is happening. It will impact on psychological activities necessary for daily living. These include the process of thought itself, judgement, perception and perceptional analysis. There are two types, the first being human behaviour related, the second being human condition related.

Human behaviour related psychological disturbance is associated with increases in stress, fear, pain, discomfort, anxiety, constant worry and despair. The behaviour required by the individual to deal with these feelings may result in their becoming angry and frustrated, especially if they perceive other people or circumstances as hindering their recovery or success. Such anger can lead to the individual feeling that it is absolutely necessary to attack the source of their frustration, be it someone else, an institution or organization, or themselves. The longer the cause of the psychological disturbance persists, the more likelihood there is of PE occurring. The significance of these types of PE for nurses is that the cause of the behaviour can often be clearly identified and, as such, dealt with either before the PE occurs, or at worst, be built into both the intervention and resolution phases of AIRS.

Human condition related psychological disturbance is associated with illness phenomena, be it physical or mental. In this case the illness itself brings about an alteration in the ability of the individual to think clearly. Any form of mental illness may fall into this category, though those which are more likely to do so are discussed below. Physical conditions where there are related psychological problems, such as toxic confusional states, the dementias, head injuries, detoxification programmes, and those requiring neuro-surgical interventions, are part of this group. There are a smaller number of iatrogenic, or doctor-induced, situations, such as drug interactions, post-anaesthesia disorientation and inappropriate interventions generally, which may also be grouped here. The significance of these types of PE for nurses is that the cause of the PEs generated by these disturbances cannot clearly be identified and consequently alternative interventions must be used within AIRS.

There are times when such differences in the cause of behaviours generating a PE are far less easy to categorize. Certain cultures and peoples see their relationships differently to others, and this can have an effect on their relationships with people outside their culture. Relationships between males and females in many parts of the world are different to those experienced by Western societies. Failure by the healthcare worker to adhere to accepted rules and practices may well generate anger and insult, which in turn may bring about an assault.

Children and young people have a tendency to be far more 'up-front' than those older than themselves. It is often the case that behaviours are used as a direct response to these older expectations, so that shocking, insulting and outrageous behaviours are seen as being acceptable by the young, and unacceptable by some adults. Responding violently to an apparent insult from a young person may outwardly seem inappropriate, but can be understood more easily when one investigates the nature of inter-age relationships. Care staff, often much younger than their client groups, may behave 'badly' without any appreciation that they have done so, while older people also appear to have a tradition of belittling youth. True, the psychological disturbance generated by these examples are of the human behaviour related type, but sometimes it is impossible to identify the cause of a PE when, through a total lack of insight, it is yourself!

Other examples of the difficulties which can be experienced in trying to identify the nature or cause of psychological disturbance are found in areas such as forensic psychiatry. Here the difficulty may be about making sense of someone's behaviour after a serious PE or series of PEs. It may also be about trying to identify causative factors which pre-empt seemingly pointless violence or aggression. Trying to establish whether someone is pretending to be mentally ill, or if they truly have such problems, is thankfully the task of experienced practitioners, yet all too often, following attacks on members of the healthcare professions, people ask the same question, 'Was it done on purpose?' The answer here is not really relevant, the fact is that it did take place and may take place once again. The degree of psychological disturbance experienced by the client will be one of the sole determinants in deciding what to do about this situation.

Acting-out behaviours also provide healthcare workers with difficulties. These are usually associated with adolescent development, and certainly within psychiatry the tradition of units and care teams specifically trained to work in this area is long founded. However, for the nurse working in a busy A&E department, knowing that someone else might know how to deal effectively with the situation of suddenly being confronted by a young girl brandishing a knife and demanding instant attention, is of little real help. Knowing that there may be a degree of psychological disturbance may be of some use, but knowing what causes it may be singularly more useful than anything. The reason for this is simple. If the nurse can readily identify that certain responses fit into the framework of the girl's needs better than others, it makes sense to use them. If the nurse knows that the girl's requirements stem from human behaviour, rather than human condition needs, simply responding to the requests for instant attention might resolve the immediate crisis. If, however, the nurse tries to reason with the girl in these circumstances, which she might decide to do if the disturbance were generated by human condition related disturbance, she has a good chance of being attacked.

Unfortunately for the nurse, the girl may be experiencing both human and condition related disturbance. This is discussed in more depth in Chapter 11, but the combination of developmental issues, drug or alcohol abuse, human needs and acting-out behaviour is extremely complex. Certainly, responding directly to the girl's needs would be the safest option. However, it is the ability of the nurse to make these decisions quickly which is important here.

At-risk groups

Part of the process of undertaking an assessment of someone at the beginning of a PE is having some understanding of their history, their general presentation and their motives. Being able to establish whether a client is suffering from human related psychological disturbance, or a condition related one, is of considerable importance. For the first it is likely that the cause can be identified, in the second it is less likely. In the assessment of the motives for a PE this therefore might determine the nature and style of the intervention used, and to some degree resolution expectations. However, as with the young girl in the A&E department example, it is likely that the two categories will overlap each other. The likelihood of one being the sole reason for the PE is very slim, but being able to identify the significantly dominant one is of prime importance.

As already said, anyone may suffer psychological disturbance. Within the human related group this is more so the case, than the condition related. It is perhaps this second group which is the most difficult for healthcare workers to understand. While not wishing to identify certain key diagnoses as being more at risk than others, there are certainly some client groups which, because of the severity of the psychological disturbance they experience, are more likely to find themselves in situations which may develop into PEs. Both ICD-10-CM and DSM-IV (1994) multiaxial systems used for classifying mental disorders, have plenty of examples of diagnoses in which aggression and violence may be present. However, within the context of this chapter it is more important to consider the at-risk groups, rather than the specific diagnosis. Individual motivation for violence will be as varied as the people who use it, while the trends experienced by certain groups tend to be more repeatable.

Childbirth

It may seem a strange group of people to begin with but pregnant mothers can get pretty aggressive! Any midwife will tell you of incidents where mothers giving birth suddenly become both verbally and physically violent as the birth progresses. However, it is not this group that concerns us here. Illingworth (1989) describes a study investigating the emotional state of mothers during the first three months after the birth. The difficulties associated with depression and feelings of self-harm were common to many. Significantly, Illingworth states that the 98 health visitors involved in the study found the information about mothers' emotional states useful, implying that they were unaware of them beforehand. This raises questions about the health care workers working with client groups for whom they have lead responsibility, but with whom they do not have either the time or the opportunity to assess degrees of psychological disturbance.

While it is not suggested here that new mothers are prone to PEs, there is some evidence to show that the high levels of stress that having a baby brings about may well put them more at risk.

Children and young people

Most of us are familiar with the comments made by most parents at some time during their children's early life – 'He is just out of control', 'Doesn't do a thing we ask' or 'What can you expect, they are only kids!' These statements imply behaviours which, whether we like them or not, we accept as being part of growing up, and tolerate because we feel that they are only transitory. These behaviours include recklessness, lack of judgement, aggressiveness, destructiveness, intolerance and many more apparently anti-social alternatives (Waszak 1992). Strange that the same behaviours exhibited by so called grownups cause us far more concern! However, the problems faced by young people may be complicated further by psychological disturbance. Muscari (1992) considers acting-out behaviours associated with adolescence as being difficult for nurses to deal with if they do not have psychiatric skills.

These behaviours in themselves may not be true psychological disturbance, more developmental, but, as Valente (1992) shows, such behaviours may develop far beyond the boundaries, even of the excepted norms of acting-out. Self-destructiveness, intended self-injury, self-poisoning and other potentially fatal activities undertaken by adolescents in the survey carried out by Hawton and Fagg (1992) would indicate that effective interventions in such PEs are of major concern. With suicide being the third leading cause of adolescent death the necessity for nurses to be able to use a framework such as

AIRS to help construct and implement appropriate responses to such PEs has to be a priority (Valente 1989). In cases where the individual has already come into contact with healthcare professionals, and is receiving help on an outpatient basis, there is evidence to show that without active follow-up this group soon becomes noncompliant with treatment and therapy programmes (Trautman *et al.* 1993). This would suggest that assertive outreach and accurate assessments are crucial activities for nurses working with this group.

Those experiencing sexual difficulties

Of course not all PEs involving children and adolescents result in their injuring themselves. Burgess and Hartman (1992) describe the difficulties of aggression towards others which is of a sexual nature. Learning to deal with sexual feelings and responses is a key component in growing up, but mixed with other mental health problems they can become intolerable for the individual experiencing them. Such responses, while not necessarily occurring in the presence of healthcare professionals, may certainly be the motivation behind other aggressive behaviours, themselves being analysed during another PE.

However, it is not only young people who suffer from sexual disturbances which may lead to a PE. The very nature of the sexual drive means that people experience strong emotions, feelings and behaviour dominating motivational impulses. Whether this constitutes a human related psychological disturbance, or a condition related one is difficult to judge, and may indeed be both. From a condition related point of view it is perhaps worth noting that those for whom mental health problems generate sexual dissonance between reality and thought, the possibility of a violent response becomes a greater possibility. If a person truly believes that they are sexually admired by others, and attempts to indulge in passionate activities, rejection will be very difficult for them to deal with. Equally, the person who believes that others are going to sexually abuse or even rape them will react violently to those they believe to be their intended attackers. Such delusions can lead to serious harm befalling both client and healthcare worker alike, but ordinary, innocent bystanders may also be at some risk. Having some understanding of the clients' main delusional content is a key factor in learning how to approach and relate to such clients. If a PE ensues from such encounters it will be this knowledge which will inform the AIRS framework in successfully dealing with the event.

Sexual delusions are not the only cause of sexuality motivated disturbance. Coming to terms with one's feelings about others, being rejected and the resultant anger it may cause, are difficulties faced by many. In reality these are human related psychological disturbances. Smith (1992) identifies specific problems for homosexual clients who feel less understood by their carers than other client groups, while Hall (1994) sees the contribution of alcohol to the sexual problem facing lesbians as being a major factor influencing their behaviour, and indeed total health experience. Though not always a sexually related condition AIDS patients too may also experience anger and bitterness as a neuropsychiatric complication. This in turn can lead to behaviours which place healthcare workers at risk of attack (Flaskerud 1987).

Generally speaking this at-risk group, i.e. those people with sexual difficulties, are a minority group, who fall into the human related psychological disturbance category. As such the nurse is in a better position to determine the cause of violent and aggressive responses within the assessment phase of AIRS and thus bring such PEs more quickly to the resolution phase. Difficulty will arise in the support phase as often these are subject areas that clients are unwilling or embarrassed to talk about. Obviously the nurse has to ensure a balance between resolving and supporting an immediate PE and helping the client confront these issues in subsequent on-going crisis intervention or psychosocial counselling. The self-harming client, especially those who self-mutilate, will need personal space and more time to resolve the PE than those attacking others for their feelings (see Chapter 5).

Drug and alcohol detoxification

This group is discussed in detail in Chapter 11, but must also be included here as they constitute a major group of at-risk clients. As will be seen it is not just those who are undergoing treatment or therapy for their addictions that are likely to generate a PE, but from a condition related disturbance point of view, those who are undergoing detoxification programmes may react violently to their withdrawal symptoms, and are therefore more of interest here.

Detoxification programmes themselves are usually carefully administered, demand the involvement and collaboration of the client and use good communication and support mechanisms to maintain them. Medication is usually used to help the client cope with both the psychological and physical responses to drug withdrawal. However, the experiences of these clients sometimes borders on the psychotic, and it is in situations like these that the potential for a violent or self-harming PE is increased.

Head injuries

Plylar (1989) discussed the difficulties associated with head injury patients who became agitated within an acute hospital setting. Behaviour was described that was both frightening to the nurse, and also to the relatives, friend and the clients themselves. Plyer felt that the recovery phase for these clients was misunderstood and led to confrontations between staff and patients and patients and visitors. While suggesting that appropriate pharmacological interventions were part of the therapeutic programme, Plyer placed insightful and sensitive nursing intervention high on the list of priorities for this group.

Accident and emergency settings, or surgical recovery areas, especially those dealing with both head injuries and neurosurgical interventions, represent high-risk areas for potential PEs. Nurses working in these areas need to ensure that their clinical work is fully understood by their client group, and in particular their motivation for carrying out the work they are doing. Plyer showed that nurses who spent time explaining their actions fully to their clients were less at risk of attack, while studies of communication and violence generally would tend to support this (see Chapter 6).

Confusional states

Any condition which brings about an alteration in the internal environment of the brain, resulting in the individual having an inability to make sense of their world is regarded as a confusional state. They may be acute, or chronic and can vary from extreme responses to constipation, where toxins are reabsorbed in the bowel and eventually interfere with cortical synapses, to the chronic problems associated with some head injuries. Confusional states are often found as an overlay for dementia, where the primary problem is not one of confusion, but disorientation. Confusion may also be an accompaniment to illnesses and conditions characterized by high temperatures, including many of the so-called childhood conditions such as measles and chicken-pox. The sufferer may experience hallucinations, altered states of awareness, mood fluctuations and, depending on the severity of the condition, altered levels of consciousness.

Nurses, and for that matter carers, looking after this particular client group are at risk only because of the sufferers' inability to make sense of themselves and their surroundings. In a sense it is the interface between reality and fantasy, what is real and what is not. When the two conflict, the danger begins to increase, and when the carer is not in a position to predict the changes in the sufferer's behaviour accurately, the possibility of a PE occurring also increases.

These are many condition related psychological disturbances. However, they represent a very extreme group. The nurse must always be aware that this group of people are far more unpredictable than most others. They tend to do normal things, but out of context (those who carry out unusual or bizarre behaviours are more likely to be in the head injury group). They are just as prone to aggressive behaviours as they are to non-aggressive ones. The mother who is suddenly confronted by her darling 12-year-old daughter, who appears to have turned into the main character in a horror movie and is attempting to smash her way out of the bedroom window, can take solace from the fact that the child had a very high temperature, and once it has subsided will return to her usual state once again. So to the nurse confronted by an elderly client apparently trying to pull the hair from the nurse's scalp, hurling abuse and threatening to fall out of bed. The nurse will know that her patient is also unwell, but might not be so tolerant of her client as the mother of her daughter. Both sufferers have confusional states, the first resulting from an increase in circulating toxins as a result of the body trying to deal with the measles, the second, an increase of toxins caused because the elderly man, suffering Alzheimer's disease, was disoriented for so long he failed to answer the call to stool, did not go to the toilet for several days and became very constipated.

In both cases medical treatment will bring about a reduction in confusion. Sadly in the second case it will not reverse the condition prompting the disorientation, and therefore this client will remain constantly at risk of perpetuating further PE behaviour. However, accurate assessment of changes in client behaviour should reduce the possibility of the hair pulling PE, even if it cannot prove totally effective against the sudden, spontaneous responses of aggression which may occur with the elderly mentally ill (Ekman *et al.* 1991).

The elderly

One group, who by definition, are at risk are the elderly, and in particular the elderly mentally ill. Not only does this group have to contend with the difficulties of old age, and possible physical infirmity, but they also have the added problems associated with mental ill health and condition related psychological disturbance. Whall *et al.* (1992) carried out a survey of the disruptive behaviours of elderly nursing home residents and found, amongst many others, that the most common were hitting, slapping, verbally aggressive remarks, screaming, property destruction and self-injury. Having to contend with the difficulties associated with confusion and disorientation, i.e. not being able to make any sense of what is being said or happening to you, or making the wrong sense, are disturbing perceptual, intellectual and emotional configurations for anyone to have to deal with. They leave the individual vulnerable at a time when they are least equipped to be able to deal with it. Rossby *et al.* (1992) found similar results, while Ryden and Feldt (1992) identified goal-directed care as the method for overcoming the aggression found within the same client group.

Similar recommendations were made by Herz *et al.* (1992) who studied the restlessness inherent in clients diagnosed as suffering from Alzheimer's disease. Although this study was in effect a drug-related random control trial the authors found that the restlessness associated with the condition was a significant contributor to the aggressiveness in the relationship between the clients and the carers. Ekman *et al.* (1991) felt that some of the difficulties for this group lay with the inability to communicate effectively, and certainly for the nurse trying to diffuse a possible aggressive PE this has to be taken into consideration.

However, there is a far more insidious and dangerous side to the PEs involving the elderly. Many people associate aggressive incidents, violent PEs and unprovoked attacks with some aspects of the elderly mentally ill client group, but self-harm in the elderly remains a constant concern. Deliberate non-compliance has been shown to be a big factor in the suicide rates of this group (Meisekothen 1993). Indirect self-destructive behaviours (ISDBs) cause many more deaths than direct methods, yet Meisekothen argues that they are very rarely taken seriously, ignored or misinterpreted. For nurses caring for the elderly mentally ill, especially within a community setting, this must form a significant factor within the AIRS assessment framework.

Receiving care in the community

The risks taken by many healthcare professionals working within a community environment are sometimes considered to be too severe to be tolerated. Certainly those individuals who suffer illnesses which cause continuous or considerable pain, for whom symptoms are both disturbing and disorientating, and where support from a carer is difficult to sustain, have a greater potential for some form of PE. While there is always the possibility of attacks against others (see Chapter 6), the difficulty with this client group is that they may be a danger to themselves.

Feeling that you are of no value to anyone, living in constant pain, seeing loved ones giving up their lives to care for you, is both dehumanizing and demoralizing. For many the only option becomes suicide, and the community care worker has to be diligent in spotting those who are at risk. There is no easy formula, though an in-depth knowledge of the client/patient is crucial to making any assessment of risk. Relationships that are developed over time are more likely to reveal the secret worries and fears of the client, while working with the carers and relatives will also bring more information to bear on the individual's state of mind.

The object of community life for those who suffer long-term illness is to enable them to have the opportunity to lead as normal a lifestyle as they can. The truth is that this just is not possible in so many cases. The extremes of illness and disturbance suffered by many mean that any relationship with normality is purely incidental. Every attempt has to be made to try to ensure that those most at risk are given the right amount of support, and resources are made available as a consequence of the healthcare worker's assessments. Incidents such as the Clunis affair (DoH 1994), where an individual with a mental health problem living in the community stabbed an innocent bystander to death in a public underground, are extreme, but they highlight the necessity for people to accept and maintain responsibility for clients at risk. Adopting keyworker type roles are crucial to this approach, and engender professional roles which incorporate spending time with clients as a method of getting to know them properly (Davis 1991).

Healthcare workers cannot afford to take risks themselves, but as we have already discussed in Chapter 6 being a community worker has its own set of risks. Part of it certainly rests with the client group, but some of the risks rest with the practices of community healthcare workers themselves. Attending people in their own homes is a risk in itself, yet very few community workers carry bleep or alarm systems. At the very least the worker ought to have a method of summoning support or assistance. A reliance on 'borrowing' the client's or the next-door neighbour's, telephone is rather outdated to say the least. In certain circumstances it is also more appropriate that community workers visit certain clients with a professional partner, or team member, as a form of backup or support. Attacks on community workers are not uncommon, and while such attacks occur it seems nonsensical for healthcare workers not to try to protect themselves and their clients from harm.

Those receiving treatment

You might think this an odd at-risk group – after all most of us at some time or another receive some form of treatment. True, but in some cases the treatment does not work as it should, and the condition suffered is worsened. In some cases responses to treatment can generate problems worse than the original condition (Valente and Saunders 1989). Iatrogenic conditions, or those brought about by medical intervention, may also generate alterations in mental awareness. Hawthorne and Lacey (1992) describe the study of a lady suffering from bulimia who developed severe disturbance following drug therapy. Self-cutting, violence, paranoid ideation and intense suicidal thoughts characterized this particular case. These are not symptoms associated with bulimia, but more the depression which accompanies it. However, the responses in this particular case were extreme, and the therapy itself may have contributed to the disturbance.

Mental health problems

In this group it is possible to include those suffering from learning difficulties as well as those with mental illness, and those who experience both (Jawed *et al.* 1993, Lovell and Reiss 1993). The link between psychological disturbance and mental health difficulties is obvious, but it is wrong to assume that the presence of one implies the presence of the other. It is also untrue to suggest that, because an individual is experiencing mental health problems, they are also likely to generate a PE.

There are those who are more at risk than others; however, providing a list of the so-called at risk diagnosis is an inappropriate way of looking at the group. What is important here is the degree of psychological disturbance being experienced by each individual client. While it is true to say that someone who is experiencing paranoid or extremely irrational thoughts of suspicion may be more at risk of a violent PE, there are always going to be clients who cope with these thoughts and feelings far better than others. The amount of insight the individual has, the type of support offered by the care team, the relationship with key workers or primary nurses, the nature and appropriateness of the treatment programme, will all play a part in the clinical presentation. The nurse's ability to undertake and act upon accurate predication of rapid mood changes and the detection of alterations in general mental state are just as crucial in heading off a potential violent incident, as are the client's symptoms. It is therefore not the clinical diagnosis alone which is a determinant factor, but the individual client's response to that diagnosis (Ward 1992).

The likelihood of a PE increases as the degree of disturbance does. It is the client's response to the disturbance which is important, as is the nurse's ability to detect the changes taking place and act accordingly. Panic attacks are a classic example of this situation. The client will present features of the condition in an obvious way, yet if the nurse dismisses them as childish or inappropriate the result may well be a very serious PE (Braverman 1990, Tommasini and Federici 1992). Similarly, the presence of hallucinations and delusions may increase the possibility of a PE, but if the nurse is able to recognize the presence of these phenomena and act in a dignified and understanding way towards the individual who is experiencing them such situations may be averted.

There is no difference in the feelings associated with fear, stress and panic for someone who has a mental illness or is severely mentally handicapped in some way, than there is for a person who has neither. The experience of fear will be the significant factor, not the presence of mental illness. In fact in some situations the experience of fear may be reduced for the client with a mental illness or learning disability as they may fail to recognize the dangers inherent in a prevailing situation. Harris (1993) undertook a survey of aggressive behaviour among people with learning disabilities in one UK health district and discovered that there was a very low threat of violence towards others, and the group generally were regarded as being relatively easy to manage. The implication here is that this group tend to be more of a danger to themselves, and that thoughtful nursing intervention can diffuse PEs relatively quickly.

Major considerations for nurses working with this at-risk group are the perceived levels of stress being exhibited, anger towards self and others, the degree of unpredictableness exhibited, alterations in mental awareness and concentration, levels of irritability, tolerance, and even consciousness. Knowledge of past behaviours, and in particular the responses to stress usually adopted by the client, the learnt responses to frustration, their capacity for disruptive behaviour and their stress tolerance levels are all major components in the assessment of this group.

Whether these psychological disturbances are as a result of human related or condition related phenomena is difficult to determine as the two appear to interact with each other. What is definite is that the nurse must use those elements of the clients' presentation that will enable him/her to predict the possibility of a PE. Knowing possible causes of behavioural changes may allow the nurse to head off the PE, but if there is a clearer appreciation of the difficulties such clients face because of the disturbance then sensitive interactions can be constructed which have a similar, resolving, effect.

Conclusion

This chapter has explored the issues related to psychological disturbance and their effects upon the individual's ability to cope with stress, frustration and anger. While it is generally agreed that the group who are most at risk of psychological disturbance are those experiencing mental health problems, it is not agreed that this group are the only ones at risk of generating PEs.

The nature of the disturbance, whether it be human related or condition related was discussed, as a method of predicting the possibility of a PE. The cause of the disturbance might lead to a greater understanding of the client's condition and as such give some degree of insight into how to deal with a potential PE should it erupt. However, health status generally was seen as indicating an individual's potential for violent responses, either to life situations, or intellectual and emotional ones.

The use of AIRS as a tool for assessment of such predicting factors is mentioned several times throughout the chapter, yet in truth AIRS is limited here to reminding the nurse that the assessment needs to be undertaken. What this chapter demonstrates is that there are at-risk groups, and, yes, they can be identified, but what is more important is that the nurse looks at each client on an individual basis, and not simply by virtue of the clinical diagnosis. In a sense the key issue here is the nursing, and not the medical diagnosis. The medical diagnosis will tell the nurse what is wrong with the client. This will remain unchanged throughout the course of the illness or condition. The nursing diagnosis will tell the nurse how the client is coping with what is wrong. It will change as the client responds, both to him/herself and to the input from others. It is this changing pattern of accurate nursing diagnosis which provides the nurse with the key to potential PEs, and it should be used to develop both the interventions and the resolution and support strategies needed to increase the client's own coping mechanisms (Ward 1992).

References

American Psychiatric Association (1994). *Diagnostic and Statistical Manual of Mental Disorders*, 4th edn. The American Psychiatric Association, Washington DC.

Braverman, B. G. (1990). Calming the patient with panic disorder. *Nursing*, **20**(1):32.

Burgess, A. W. and Hartman, C. R. (1992). Nursing interventions with children and adolescents experiencing sexually aggressive responses. In P. West *et al.* (eds), *Psychiatric and Mental Health Nursing with Children and Adolescents*, Aspen Pubs, Gaithersburg.

Davis, A. J. (1991). Dilemmas in alternative care settings. *Western Journal of Nursing Research*, **13**(5):650–2.

Department of Health (1994). *The Report of the Enquiry into the Care and Treatment of Christopher Clunis*. HMSO, London.

Ekman, S., Norberg, A., Viitanen, M. and Winblad, B. (1991). Care of demented patients with severe communication problems. *Scandinavian Journal of Caring Sciences*, **5**(3):163– 70.

Finnema, E. J., Dassen, T. and Halfens, R. (1994). Aggression in psychiatry: a qualitative study focusing in the characterization and perception of patient aggression by nurses working on psychiatric wards. *Journal of Advanced Nursing,* **19**:1088–95.

Flaskerud, J. H. (1987). AIDS: neuropsychiatric complications. *Journal of Psychosocial Nursing and Mental Health Services,* **25**(12):17–20, 35, 37.

Hall, J. M. (1994). Lesbians recovering from alcohol problems: an ethnographic study of health care experiences. *Nursing Research,* **43**(4):238–45.

Harris, P. (1993). The nature and extent of aggressive behaviour amongst people with learning difficulties (mental handicap) in a single health district. *Journal of Intellectual Disabilities Research,* **37**(3):221–42.

Hawthorne, M. E. and Lacey, J. H. (1992). Severe disturbance occurring during treatment for depression of a bulimic patient. *Journal of Affective Disorders,* **26**(3):205–7.

Hawton, K. and Fagg, J. (1992). Deliberate self-poisoning and self injury in adolescents: a study of characteristics and trends in Oxford. *British Journal of Psychiatry,* **161**:816– 23.

Heron, J. (1977). *Carthasis in Human Development,* Human Potential Research Project, University of Surrey, Guildford.

Herz, L. R., Volicer, L., Ross, V. and Rheaume, Y. (1992). A single case-study method for treating restlessness in patients with Alzheimer's disease. *Hospital and Community Psychiatry,* **43**(7):720–4.

Holmes, T. and Rahe, R. (1967). The social readjustment rating scale. *Journal of Psychosomatic Research,* **11**:213.

Illingworth, C. (1989). The emotional state of mothers in the first three months after the birth of their baby. *Health Visitor,* **62**(11):340–2.

Jahoda, M. (1958). *Current Concepts of Positive Mental Health.* Basic Books Publishers, New York.

Jawed, S. H., Krishman, V. H., Prasher, V. P. and Corbett, J. A. (1993). Worsening of pica as a symptom of depressive illness in a person with severe mental handicap. *British Journal of Psychiatry,* **162**:835–7.

Lovell, R. W. and Reiss, A. L. (1993). Dual diagnosis: psychiatric disorders in developmental disabilities. *Paediatric Clinics of North America,* **40**(3):579–92.

Meisekothen, L. M. (1993). Noncompliance in the elderly: a pathway to suicide. *Journal of American Academic Nurse Practitioner,* **5**(2):67–72.

Muscari, M. E. (1992). The 'acting-out' adolescent: identification and management. *Paediatric Nursing*, **18**(4):362–6.

Newnes, C. (1993). What is mental health? *Clinical Psychology Forum*, **51**:32–3.

Newnes, C. (1994). Defining mental health? *Nursing Times*, **90**(19):46.

Plylar, P. A. (1989). Management of the agitated and aggressive head injury patient in an acute hospital setting. *Journal of Neuroscience Nursing*, **21**(6):353–6.

Rossby, L., Beck, C. and Heacock, P. (1992). Disruptive behaviours of cognitively impaired nursing home residents. *Archives of Psychiatric Nursing*, **6**(2):98–107.

Ryden, M. B. and Feldt, K. S. (1992). Goal-directed care: caring for aggressive nursing home residents with dementia. *Journal of Gerontological Nursing*, **18**(11):35–42.

Smith, G.B. (1992). Nursing care challenges: homosexual psychiatric patients. *Journal of Psychosocial Nursing and Mental Health Services*, **30**(12):15–21, 37–8.

Swanson, J. W., Holzer, C. E., Ganju, V. K. and Jono, R. T. (1990). Violence and psychiatric disorder in the community: evidence from the epidemiologic catchment area surveys. *Hospital and Community Psychiatry*, **41**:761–9.

Tommasini, N. R. and Federici, C. M. (1992). Recognition of panic disorder in the emergency department. *Journal of Emergency Nursing*, **18**(4):319–28.

Trautman, P. D., Stewart, N. and Morishima, A. (1993). Are adolescent suicide attempters noncompliant with outpatient care? *Journal of American Child and Adolescent Psychiatry*, **32**(1):89–94.

Valente, S. M. (1989). Adolescent suicide: assessment and intervention. *Child and Adolescent Psychiatric Mental Health Nursing*, **21**:34–9.

Valente, S. M. (1992). Nursing interventions with children and adolescents experiencing self-destructive tendencies. In P. West *et al.* (eds), *Psychiatric and mental health nursing with children and adolescents*, Aspen Pubs, Gaithersburg.

Valente, S. M. and Saunders, J. M. (1989). Dealing with serious depression in cancer patients. *Nursing*, **19**(2):44– 7.

Ward, M. F. (1992) *The Nursing Process in Psychiatry*, 2nd edn. Churchill Livingstone, Edinburgh.

Waszak, L. C. (1992). Nursing interventions with children and adolescents experiencing conduct difficulties. In P. West *et al.* (eds), *Psychiatric and Mental Health Nursing with Children and Adolescents*. Aspen Pubs, Gaithersburg.

Whall, A. L., Gillis, G. L., Yankou, D., Booth, D. E. and Beel-Bates, C. A. (1992). Disruptive behaviour in elderly nursing home residents: a survey of nursing staff. *Journal of Gerontological Nursing*, 18(10):13–17.

Winger, J., Schim, V. and Stewart, D. (1987). Aggressive behaviour in long term care. *Journal of Psychosocial Nursing and Mental Health Services*, 25:28–33.

Suggested reading

Brant, B. A. and Osgood, N. J. (1990). The suicidal patient in long term care institutions. *Journal of Gerontological Nursing*, 16(2):15–18, 36–7. (Provides a good backdrop to the problems associated with this at-risk group and explores the nursing issues of assessment and intervention.)

Puskar, K., Hoover, C. and Miewald, C. (1992). Suicidal and nonsuicidal coping methods of adolescents. *Perspectives in Psychiatric Care*, 28(2):15–20. (This study considers the difference in the two coping strategies and offers clues for effective nursing assessments.)

Rosenthal, T. T. and McGuinness, T. M. (1986). Dealing with delusional patients: discovering the distorted truth. *Issues in Mental Health Nursing*, 8(2):143–54. (This study describes how certain clients with delusions view their world, using grounded theory to generate five different type of delusion. The process of decoding client experiences is invaluable for nurses seeking to understand the precipitants for delusion motivated PEs.)

Smith, R. G., Iwata, B. A., Vollmer, T. R. and Zarcone, J. R. (1993). Experimental analysis and treatment of multiple controlled self-injury. *Journal of Applied Behavioural Analysis*, 26(2):183–96. (A study of three people with profound learning disabilities who continuously engage in self-injurious behaviours. Assessment and intervention issues are discussed.)

11

Emergencies associated with drugs and alcohol

Introduction

A psychiatric emergency may happen to anyone, but as we have seen from Chapter 10 some people are more at risk than others. Being at risk does not mean that they are definitely going to experience such an event. For example, a racing driver could be said to be in a dangerous occupation where, because of the speeds being driven and the competitive nature of the sport, the possibility of a serious accident was greatly increased. However, it does not mean that the racing driver will definitely have a serious accident. Similarly, being at risk of a PE does not mean that a person will necessarily do so, but it does mean that their chances of experiencing one are increased either because of their personal circumstances, or more likely, because of psychological disturbance.

In the same way that the racing driver takes precautions to ensure that s/he does not crash, so there appears to be a sort of control mechanism inside of us which warns us of impending danger. The warning signals can be biological or psychological, but they have the effect of making us aware of our emotional state. In most cases we respond positively to these, but there are occasions when we do not heed the warning, and that is when a PE is more likely to occur.

Certain forces can interrupt our appreciation of what is happening to us. The illnesses and conditions described in Chapter 10 are examples of these forces, all having some bearing upon our ability to deal effectively with what is going on around us. The degree of psychological disturbance we experience may well be the factor which determines the potential for a PE, with the higher levels being more prone than the lower ones.

There is one at-risk group not discussed in Chapter 10 which needs to be considered in more detail. Racing drivers need to be alert and highly responsive, with a reasonable splattering of good judgement thrown in. The one thing they would not do is consume alcohol just before a race, and the possibility of being drunk on the starting grid is beyond comprehension. The same applies to the taking of any other mind-altering drugs. The reason for this is simple, drugs and alcohol act upon the central nervous system and have a direct impact upon intellectual activities, thus diluting the very qualities required to be a successful racing driver. However, drugs and alcohol can have serious effects upon human behaviour which may result in the user, or others, being more at risk. It is because the desired effects of these drugs is to alter the way the user feels, responds and perceives, that the risk factor is increased. Further alterations in mood, perception and judgement only compound the problem.

The effects of drugs and alcohol

To be able to appreciate why this is a special group it is important to consider what happens to a person when they consume substances which alter the way their brain works.

Some drugs act to suppress the central nervous system; these include alcohol; solvents, such as glues and gases; hypnosedatives, such as barbiturates; sedatives, and minor tranquillizers. Used in moderation, or for medically prescribed purposes, the tranquillizing and sedative effects of these drugs enable people to become more relaxed, and experience things in a less threatening way. Used to extremes, they may generate hostility and anger as the individual becomes more disinhibited.

Other drugs stimulate the central nervous system, thus emulating the effects of the sympathetic nervous system in preparing the body to deal with difficult or dangerous situations. These drugs include amphetamines and cocaine, and its smokable form, 'crack'. These drugs produce physiological arousal, accompanied by exhilaration and a general sense of well-being. Continuous use can produce sleeplessness, paranoia, agitation confusion and mood swings.

A third group, about which the specific cortical effects are known in different degrees, are the hallucinogens, or 'psyche-delics'. These drugs alter the individual's perceptional abilities and include lysergic acid diethylamide (LSD) and cannabis. The user's mood tends to influence the effects of these drugs, with both the social setting and expectations having similar impact. Perceptional distortions occur accompanied by height-ened awareness of body function. In the case of LSD, and other naturally occurring substances such as 'magic mushrooms', or hallucinogenic mushrooms, flashbacks may occur. These are often the experience of reliving the bad effects which happen during the taking of the drug – known as a 'bad trip'. They may leave the individual distressed and frightened.

The final group are the opiates, or narcotic analgesics. They have considerable medical use, both as analgesics, cough suppressants and anti-diarrhoea agents. They include opium, heroin and morphine, with most people being aware of their more common medically prescribed member, codeine. When used for non-prescribed purposes they are very quick acting central nervous system depressants. The user becomes drowsy and reaches a state of contentment. The more the drug is used, the more is required to produce the necessary state of well-being. This tolerance may result in overdoses, or mixing drugs, which may have more serious consequences for the user, including coma and death.

For the alcohol user the main objective appears to be to reach a state of well-being sometimes referred to as the 'dizzy and delightful' stage. This includes a reduction in personal inhibi-tions, feeling more confident and generally achieving a state of well-being. However, as more alcohol is consumed the drinker progresses into the 'drunk' stage, with a general reduction in judgement and physical and social competence. More alcohol will result in the 'dead drunk' stage, the drinker staggering and becoming totally disinhibited and socially incompetent. Violence and aggression may be experienced towards others both during the drunk and dead drunk stages, though people may be irritated by the drinker during his/her 'dizzy' phase. The final stage of intoxification is the 'dead' stage. The drinker falls and becomes unconscious, suffocating on their own vomit, stops breathing or suffers exposure and hypothermia.

With very few exceptions the drugs identified above may precipitate a PE while they are being used or acquired, or once they are withdrawn. In other words, after prolonged use of drugs the user will experience serious physical, emotional and psychological responses if they do not continue to use it. During detoxification or withdrawal programmes the client is likely to increase their potential for a violent, possibly self-harming PE quite considerably.

While the behaviour of the intoxicated, or 'under the influence', individual is of significance to nurses and healthcare professionals, so too is that of the individual who has become addicted to drugs or alcohol. As the psychological dependence is reinforced and ultimately replaced in intensity by the physical one, so the users' desire for the substance they are abusing becomes more intense. The psychological dependence is the craving for the effects of the drug, while the physical one is the biological demand for the substance to be present in the body. These demands become irresistible, and place the abuser in a position where s/he has to get their drug to be able to survive. Eventually finding, acquiring and using the drug becomes their main daily preoccupation, to the exclusion of all else.

Healthcare workers are therefore faced with three groups of individuals who may be using drugs and/or alcohol, each of whom may present with a separate set of demands, each of whom are more at risk of a PE, but for different reasons. The casual users, the drunk in the A&E department, the client returning from the pub after a few drinks, despite being on psychotropic medication, the cannabis user who has just been beaten up in the street because he failed to recognize the dangers to himself, present an immediate threat, both to themselves, and the healthcare worker. The addict, chronic abuser or 'alcoholic' presents a more complicated picture, because in the craving to acquire the substance they need they may abscond, thus placing themselves even more at risk, or demand with threats of violence, the substances they need. It is not uncommon for addicts to enter A&E departments with hand guns and knives and hold nurses hostage until they are given the keys to drug cupboards. And finally, the third group, more likely to be in-patients than the other two groups, consists of those receiving support during a withdrawal programme. This group is more at risk during the first week after withdrawal of the drug, especially if withdrawal delirium (delirium tremens or 'DTs') or alcoholic hallucinosis accompanies the general withdrawal symptoms.

Drugs, alcohol and behaviour

As already described, drugs tend to alter the way in which the brain works, thereby allowing the user to access thoughts, feelings, beliefs and personal competencies that they might not normally do. Inevitably, as the individual changes his/her thought process, so his or her behaviour will alter, but while what is thought is only limited by the person's imagination, behaviour is limited to that which already exists. So, a person who is drunk and demanding attention will not invent new and entertaining behaviours to do so. S/he will shout, be abusive, throw things, and assault just the same as anybody else would. The problem is that this behaviour will not be nullified in the same way that others may. The drinker has alcohol in his blood system and it will take many hours for it to be metabolized or excreted. Consequently, a PE with a drunk is likely to last a lot longer than it might with someone else.

What behaviours might be exhibited? This will depend very much on the type of drug which has been used, but central to this theory is the significance played by the state of mind the user is in when using the drug, the company that they are in, the motivation for using the drugs and the expectation they have of using it. For example, if someone goes out for a celebratory party, then they will be in a good mood, cheerful and happy. If, during the evening they fall out with a partner, become separated from friends, begin to feel unwell, or even over-consume, then their mood will begin to change and they become more combative or defensive. The behaviour exhibited in the early stages of the evening will be very different to that of the latter.

Generally speaking those behaviours that will trouble nurses will include those where the client/patient is combative, agitated, demanding and angry. During certain stages of substance abuse some clients can become extremely suspicious of both their environment as well as the people in it. Of course, some of the behaviours exhibited by users and abusers alike will not be seen by the nurse. In the case of drugs that are taken to enhance a person's awareness of his body function, the rush of excitement these drugs initially generate, and the state of total calmness that exists for some users over several hours, will mean that they are abusing in private. These individuals are at risk of other forms of PE. As the individual begins to feel that they are capable of doing almost anything so too their judgement becomes increasingly impaired. The chances of their hurting themselves are very high, especially if they are taking drugs on their own and do not have others to look after them. Feeling that they can fly, and jumping off a tower block to experience it, would, during this stage of their 'trip', seem perfectly logical.

The behaviour changes as the public nature of the abuse changes. Hence, drinking alcohol, while being reasonably socially acceptable under most circumstances, is not necessarily acceptable once it has reached the 'dead drunk' stage. The reason is quite simple: people who have had one or two drinks tend to be quite polite and talkative, while drunks tend to threaten social order! As a consequence the more public the behaviour, the more drunk or intoxicated the individual tends to be, and the more anti-social the behaviour is becoming. Once it gets to the point where confrontation, abuse and threats of violence are used as methods of communication, the abuser has reached the end of the behavioural continuum. They have, in effect, lost control of themselves, their emotions, the psychological processes and their social performance.

Not all abusers of drugs and alcohol are at risk of experiencing a PE. For some individuals their state of mind, their ability to relate to others and the company they keep may deflect them from serious harm. For others, the behaviours of abuse will only increase the potential for a PE when, overwhelmed by the remorse and guilt generated by some drugs, they seriously consider self-harm, or even suicide as the effects of the drug wear off. Others may develop other behaviours of self-abuse which are only compounded by drug or alcohol use, and as such it may be these behaviours, and not the substance abuse, which brings them to the attention of the heathcare worker via some form of PE. Evans and Lacey (1992) describe a study which looked at the self-damaging behaviours of female alcoholics. They found that very often treatment for alcoholism was thwarted because of other impulsive behaviours, such as loss of control of eating. However, more significantly they found that three-quarters of the sample had behavioural problems, including deliberate self-harm, physical violence and self-cutting.

For care staff working with abusing clients key issues concerning the clients' motivation need to be considered. Behaviours associated with the abuse of alcohol and drugs can be more clearly understood and dealt with if the care staff are aware of them. If, however, clients hide their addictions, cravings or drug requirements, then the behaviours they exhibit can be far more difficult for staff to deal with. McMahon and Jones (1992) discuss the difficulties associated with the process of denial attributed to most alcoholics.

However, this denial is present in most people with some form of addiction. If a person comes into hospital to have investigations for heart problems, and appears to be smelling of alcohol all the time, the nurses are going to become increasingly irritated by him. If they discover that he has secreted a bottle of spirits in the toilet and is having a 'tipple' every now and again, they are going to become even more angry with him, with the likelihood of his being discharged if he does not cease his behaviour. Obviously here the behaviour was the smelling of alcohol, in itself not really a problem, but it is the implications of flouting the hospital code and invalidating costly investigations and treatments which are the issue. As we will see later the care professional's behaviour towards such clients will influence the potential for a violent PE (Gallop and Wynn 1987, Lewis and Appleby 1988).

Drugs, alcohol and the PE: care staff attitude

The result of the influence of drugs and alcohol upon the individual's thought processes, intellectual capabilities, emotional responses and general well-being, and the subsequent behaviours which they generate, will all need to be taken into consideration before making any comment about their impact upon possible PEs. Obviously the potential for a PE is increased in a great many cases, but there is a final factor to be included before discussing possible intervention options.

Care staff need to be aware of the effects they have upon all of their clients. However, for this at-risk group this knowledge could mean the difference between a successful encounter or a serious assault. As already described being aware of the nature of a person's behaviour will influence the response towards them, so if the nurse is aware that the client has a problem with drinking, this can be built into the strategies used to interact with him/her. Likewise, if the client is involved in a detoxification programme it is expected that they will experience traumatic and frightening symptomotology, and this will be reflected in the nurse's interventions. In both these situations the nurse would have some degree of control over the care environment, and might share responsibility for care with the client as and when s/he was able to assume responsibility for themselves.

What then of a situation where the client had control over the care situation, as in the case of a district nurse visiting an elderly man in his own home, finding that he is under the influence of alcohol, demanding that she share a drink with him? How does the nurse respond? Does she remonstrate with the patient, tell him he ought not drink so much, tell him that she is insulted, refuse the drink, storm out of the house? Does she do none of these except try to reason with him, still refusing to take the drink but not remonstrating with him about his own drinking? Or does she accept a small drink, stay for a short while distracting the man until he is ready to have his treatment carried out? In truth the answer is none of these, though a combination of one or two of the above may bring about a successful home visit. The fact is that in this circumstance, where the patient's behaviour is such that it places the nurse at risk if she refuses to co-operate with his wishes, the nurse is not in control, and therefore cannot dictate the style, pace and nature of their interaction.

Tmobranski (1994) discusses the process of patient–nurse negotiation and questions whether it exists as a reality within clinical practice, despite being espoused as representing good practice. She concludes that the desire to negotiate and share in decision-making has to be a personal choice, with both nurse and patient actively involved. However, she does not describe situations where the empowerment issue has been wrestled from the nurse and placed with the client. When the client assumes more control of the care environment, or the interaction, it is usually because they want something from it (Ward 1993). If one adds to that situation the fact that the client has lost some control over themselves as a result of drug- or alcohol-taking then the possibility of negotiation and shared responsibility is greatly reduced, thus putting the nurse even more at risk.

The nurse has to try to find the balance between the requirements of the therapeutic intervention, and the degree of psychological disturbance (generated by intoxification). What s/he cannot afford to do is antagonize the client, disrupt the pattern of the thought processes, or set up a situation where there are winners and losers. The nurse is the key component in the interaction. The more antagonistic s/he is towards the client the more likely is the event to escalate. The more intolerant s/he is of the client's behaviour, the more likely the client will increase the behaviour. The less the nurse reacts to the insult, abuse and general discomfort of the encounter, the more likely that no-one will be harmed.

The district nurse mentioned has to consider how important is the treatment she was about to give, and is her best course of action to get out of the house a quickly as possible, document the visit properly and discuss with her colleagues what to do next? There will be times when the medical or nursing priority has to prevail, and these are perhaps far harder issues to describe. If a drunken patient with a severe head injury is brought into an A&E department, the nurse can hardly refuse to see him because he keeps trying to maul her. She has got to act, and the manner in which she deals with this situation will ultimately have a direct bearing upon the patient's access to treatment. This is not a debate about whether both male and female nurses and care staff should allow themselves to be abused for the general good of mankind, which they obviously should not, but more about how to project a professional image when they are under extreme stress and enable the process of care to take place.

In Chapter 4 we considered the basis of intervention within a PE. Both direct and indirect actions were deemed to be of value. It was at this point that we also introduced the game plan and pointed out the necessity of making quick decisions about what to do, then seeing them through till they had been successful, or needed to be changed, again quickly, until the PE had been resolved. When dealing with clients who are drunk or intoxicated in some way these principles of action are just as important to bear in mind as at any other time, except that certain elements need to be accentuated. There must be no ambiguity between what the nurse says to the patient, and the actions which are carried out. There must be no difference in the verbal behaviour of the nurse and the non-verbal behaviour, and the use of environmental factors is of great importance.

Intervention options

The following illustrate these points.

- Try to speak plainly – use language that the client can understand.
- Use short sentences. Say what you have to say using uncomplicated and simple messages.
- Try to speak slowly – there is a tendency when feeling stressed to speak rapidly, and in a slightly higher pitched voice. Both of these hinder effective communication. The client needs to be able to hear what you are saying and make sense of it with ease, if communication is to be effective.
- Maintain good eye contact, but not to the extent that it becomes threatening.
- Stay at arm's reach from the client. If s/he moves towards you, try to move out of the way.
- Avoid touching the client if possible – obviously if a clinical procedure has to take place this will be difficult to achieve but the nurse ought to avoid trying to move or direct the client by touching.

- Try to work in pairs.
- If working in pairs is not possible, at least let another member of the team know where you are, what you are doing and with whom you are working. If clients are intoxicated, this should be recorded somewhere, and every member of the team should be aware of it.
- If one member of the team manages to develop a good relationship with the client, then it is unwise to change nurses, or introduce new care staff to the client. It can become confusing trying to make sense of who everyone is, and the confusion may lead to aggression. Where possible, restrict the number of people in contact with the client to one or two chosen staff. If, however, it is obvious that the staff selected are not getting on with the client, change the staff as soon as possible.
- This last point will obviously be a problem if there is only one member of staff, so alternatives must be found – a nurse who is finding his/her approach to an intoxicated client ineffective has to change the game plan. This may require altering the whole approach, both verbal and non-verbal, and will need to be evaluated continuously until the most effective approach is found.
- Do not get trapped in a room from which you do not have an escape route – this applies also to being manoeuvred onto a corner where furniture or the client would restrict your movement.
- Keep your hands in front of you, do not hide them behind your back – this is done for two reasons: (1) to show that you are not hiding anything from the client, and (2) to ensure that if s/he attempts to grab you, you are able to defend yourself quickly.
- Do not antagonize the client, either by actively seeking to show him/her 'who the boss is', or by using a condescending or patronizing tone of voice.
- Try to avoid disagreeing with the client. If s/he says something which is obviously wrong, but really is not important, leave it alone. If s/he says something which is important, in particular a request which cannot be complied with, find a way to deflect the request into something which can be complied with.

The last of these points needs to be considered in more detail. If a client continuously finds that every statement they make is met with disagreement and argument, they will become frustrated and angry. If there appears to be a certain amount of agreement between the client and the nurse, then this antagonism will not exist to the same extent and the possibility of a violent PE occurring may diminish. The nurse has to create the illusion of agreement, even where it does not exist. Thus, a client who asks for another drink of alcohol, would obviously benefit from a glass of water or a cup of black coffee. The game plan for the nurse is to make the connection for the client between drinking, and coffee, rather than drinking and alcohol. During the ensuing conversation, the nurse does not directly disagree with anything that the client says, thereby generating an interaction in which it appears that they are both saying the same thing, and agreeing with the client only when eventually s/he says that they would like a cup of coffee.

This is a very simple example of the technique, but the same approach can be adopted in far more complicated and dangerous situations. The important thing for the nurse to remember is that any confrontation will ultimately increase the possibility of a PE. If the confrontational element can be reduced by restructuring even the most simple of conversations held with the client, then this has to be included in the game plan. What the nurse has to remember is that the client will not respond to a reasonable request in the same way that a sober person will. Hence, there is no point in quoting rules and regulations, or pointing out the implications of their actions for others, say in the case of a client who returns drunk to a ward, making so much noise that they wake all the other clients. The client will not respond with an apology and go quietly to bed simply because the nurse has presented a logical reason for doing so, i.e. it is late and others are trying to sleep. On the contrary, the client is more likely to shout louder on the basis that they ought to have a party, and in any case, why is everyone in bed when it is so early!

If the client is using a different frame of reference for his/her relationship with the world, the nurse who is part of that world, has to adopt an appropriate response. It will need to be manufactured specifically to fit into the client's perception of what is happening, but, as the example quoted above shows, there is no reason why this response should not lead the client towards a safer and more effective set of circumstances. The nurse has to recognize the necessity to be flexible. Knowing that it is against the client's care contract to consume alcohol does not alter the fact that s/he has done it, nor does it change the fact that the nurse has got to do something about it. Telling the client that the contract has been broken will not alter the fact. Getting angry with the client because the nurse feels let down, or rejected, is not what the care programme is about. Likewise, quoting rules at someone who obviously cannot respond appropriately to them is not therapeutic.

The nurse has to consider the best options available to resolve the current situation, and this may mean bending the rules a little to do so. It certainly calls for tolerance. Allowing someone to sit up most of the night talking quietly, till they feel ready to retire is infinitely more acceptable than being assaulted. It is also more therapeutic. The next day will be the time to discuss the implications of the client's actions, not when s/he is unable to comprehend what is happening. In the same way that a PE is resolved, but the causes may sometimes remain to be tackled at a later date, so too the client who is intoxicated needs to have the immediate problem of the intoxification dealt with, leaving the far more serious causes to be dealt with at a later date.

The use of restraint

Of course, there are going to be times when the client is so disturbed that they are unable to respond to any form of reason. This may occur during a detoxification programme, either because the client's craving becomes so powerful that they can no longer resist, or because their hallucinatory and delusionary processes distort their thinking so badly. It may also occur because the client is so intoxicated that they are unable even to reason with themselves, as in the 'dead drunk' stage noted earlier. In such circumstances the nurse has to remember the first basic rule of nursing a PE - protect yourself from harm or danger. As discussed in Chapter 10, the extent of the psychological disturbance will determine the potential for a serious PE, and the same applies here, except that the cause of this condition related disturbance is either drugs or alcohol. The more disturbed the client, the greater the risk of a PE, and the greater the risk factor the greater the potential for harm, not only to the client, but also the nurse.

There are two ways that the risk factor can be reduced. The first is by removing the risk itself. This is done by recognizing the potential for a PE and undertaking precautionary interventions, such as deflecting discussions, allowing a client more freedom, spending time talking about issues important to the client, giving the client more decision-making opportunities, or just listening, thus reducing the potential. The second, restraining a client already involved in a PE, is potentially more hazardous because it is an acknowledgement of the extent to which the client has become disturbed, and therefore more difficult to reason with. The decision to restrain a client is always going to be a difficult one to make, but perhaps more so in the case of a client who is intoxicated. The client does not respond to reason, has become violent or aggressive either to themselves or others and is restrained. Then what? Simply because they are restrained does not mean they regain the access to reason. They are intoxicated and the state may continue or several hours. Do the team restrain for that period?

The problems associated with restraint were discussed in Chapter 8, but it was agreed that the main purpose of restraining a client was to protect themselves or others from serious harm, in a situation where all other interventions had failed. Certainly such an agreement also applies here. However, there are two other factors to be taken into consideration. The first has already been mentioned – the contribution of the intoxification substance to the level of psychological disturbance, and its continued impact upon the client's ability to think clearly. The second is that sometimes drug and alcohol related PEs just do not seem to have any purpose. What the restraint agreement does not take into account is that there may not have been any prior warning that a client was about to become violent or aggressive. In the case of someone presenting for treatment at an A&E department in the early hours of the morning, there will be absolutely no warning until the person arrives. In the case of a client in his own home being visited by the community nurse, the nurse will not be aware of the danger till they walk in the door. In the case of someone who is under the influence of mind-altering drugs, the attack may be the product of a totally misperceived set of thoughts, perceptions and feelings, with the victim innocent of any wrongdoing. Yet the need for restraint may be present in any one of these situations.

Care professionals need to construct strategies which include restraint procedures. Certain staff are more at risk than others, and it is these who need to ensure that restraining activities are well thought through, rehearsed and practised according to agreed principles. Recognizing that you may be attacked, or that your clients are more at risk of hurting themselves, is crucial to establishing the need for a restraining strategy. Working with clients who abuse substances is definitely one of those groups. The care team need to decide what they will achieve if they do restrain someone, how the restraining process is to be discontinued, in other words, what factors must occur for restraint to be removed, and how the effectiveness of that restraint is to be measured and evaluated. Finally, they also need to decide who is to carry out the restraint – though in the case of the spontaneous PE there may not be any choice – and what the roles of the individual team members are during the restraining process.

Grabbing hold of a person constitutes an assault, so the team have to know exactly what they are doing and why. Their actions must be in self-defence or to protect a person from obvious harm. Their actions must be seen to be relative to the amount of force necessary to reduce the harm, and the actions of all concerned must be in accordance with their agreed procedures. Most importantly of all these actions must be pre-determined. Each member of the team needs to know what to do if restraint is called for. Simply 'making it up as you go along' is both unprofessional and dangerous.

Finally, in Chapter 8, we also discussed breakaway techniques. These are particularly relevant here because they are likely to be the nurse's first line of defence against an assault from a drunken or intoxified client. They will probably need to be used in conjunction with restraint procedures, though not always. Not all clients, having made an initial assault on a member of staff, go on to require full restraint. Some become tearful and full of regret and, while still posing a threat of a further PE, are far easier to manage than those who continue to assault. The nurse has to know how to protect him/herself against drunken clients long before learning how to help the client.

Conclusion

This chapter has concentrated on the issues surrounding clients who abuse drugs, including alcohol, and become disturbed to the point where they are no longer able to respond to reason and therefore pose a threat to themselves or others. We have seen that the use of these substances may alter the user's ability to think clearly, make rational decisions, use good judgement and interact with others effectively. As a consequence the degree of psychological disturbance they experience makes them difficult clients to work with and places them at risk as far as psychiatric emergencies are concerned.

PEs involving these clients may involve harm to themselves, especially in the case of those who become morose and saddened by the substance abuse, or towards others, in the case of those that blame others for failing to see things as they do. The effects that these drugs have upon the central nervous system makes the users' behaviour somewhat predictable, but will give no indication as to the nature or target of their thoughts.

We have also considered the problems associated with detoxification programmes, though to an extent these are more controlled as both the abuser and the care team are working through a series of anticipated outcomes. These clients remain potentially susceptible to a PE, but the therapeutic environment in which they are being supported tends to reduce the risk factor slightly. Those being detoxified within their own homes pose a completely different set of problems, but here the risk may be towards their own carers, rather than healthcare professionals. The community team have a responsibility to help prepare those carers.

There is not a single set of rules for dealing with clients who abuse drugs, and then experience a PE. However, it is crucial that early detection of the possibility of such behaviours be made, with supportive and sensitive interventions being used to reduce the potential. The nurse's attitude and demeanour towards the client, both during this critical period, and later should a PE ensue, is of great importance. The nurse must be aware of their impact upon the client and try to maintain a non-threatening, value negative, stance.

These types of PEs can be extremely difficult to manage, and require skill and support from care team members. Consequently nurses should try to work in pairs, not take unnecessary chances, co-ordinate their actions, and not leave vulnerable members of the team, i.e. young females, nursing students, unqualified staff, to work on their own with this client group. A strategy must be developed to deal with all levels of interaction with those abusing drugs, and it must clearly identify the roles of individual team members. Finally, the need for restraint must be recognized, and appropriate actions be taken to ensure that its use is not abused, nor does it place clients or care staff in more danger during the psychiatric emergency.

References

Evans, C. and Lacey, J. H. (1992). Multiple self damaging behaviour among alcoholic women: a prevalence study. *British Journal of Psychiatry*, **161**:643–7.

Gallop, R. and Wynn, F. (1987). The difficult in-patient: identification and response by staff. *Canadian Journal of Psychiatry*, **32**:211–15.

Lewis, G. and Appleby, L. (1988). Personality disorder: the patient the psychiatrists dislike. *British Journal of Psychiatry*, **153**:44–9.

McMahon, J. and Jones, B. T. (1992). The change process in alcoholics: client motivation and denial in the treatment of alcoholism within the context of contemporary nursing. *Journal of Advanced Nursing*, **17**(2):173–86.

Tmobranski, P. H. (1994). Nurse–patient negotiation: assumption or reality. *Journal of Advanced Nursing*, **19**:733–7.

Ward, M. F. (1993). Communication within the psychiatric nursing process. MPhil thesis. University of East Anglia, Norwich.

Suggested reading

Gallop, R. (1992). Self destructive and impulsive behaviour in the patient with a borderline personality disorder: re-thinking hospital treatment and management. *Archives of Psychiatric Nursing,* **6**(3):178–82. (This paper considers the background to some drug and alcohol abusing clients' clinical support and offers alternatives to traditional intervention.)

Zerwekh, J. (1991). The practice of empowerment and coercion by expert public health nurses. *Image,* **24**(2):101–5. (Provides excellent information about developing relationships with difficult clients.)

12

Dealing with failure: staff support

Introduction

I can imagine the following appearing on a philosophy question paper, 'The psychiatric emergency – success or failure? Discuss'. The fact is that some people will always see any form of conflict as a failure, yet aggression itself is a naturally occurring human emotion which can provide strength and purpose. Conflict occurs as a direct response to disagreement which in turn may have an aggressive consequence. However, as we have seen throughout this book, not all PEs involve aggression, but nearly all have some measure of disagreement, and most will generate conflict as the needs of the client clash with the needs of the carer. Hence, the word failure is discussed in this chapter not in the form of judgement as to whether or not PEs should happen, but about the individuals involved and their feelings concerning their behaviour during them.

The chapter is divided into two sections. The first deals with the micro issues, in other words, how an individual is affected by their involvement in one or more PEs, and their implications for future involvement. The second deals with the macro issues, the collective impact of individuals' experiences upon the organization, and its subsequent ability to support those individuals effectively. However, to fully appreciate the effects a PE may have upon therapeutic activities, professional relationships and care performance generally, it is important to explore the broader effects associated with violence and aggression. These two sections are therefore preceded by a discussion on the relationship between the various forms of stress generated by a PE, and their relationship with the broader issues of self-efficacy, staff burnout and post-traumatic stress disorder (PTSD).

The effects of violence

A man is walking home from work. As he passes a bus stop another man steps in front of him and asks him for money. The first man refuses to give him any, and the second man hits him in the face. The people standing in the bus queue turn the other way and as the first man calls out for assistance the second man hits him again and runs away. No-one helps the first man until the assailant has disappeared, then only to ask if he is all right, which is a silly question because his mouth and nose are bleeding. The man says that he is all right, wipes his face with a handkerchief, and walks home. Once there he makes himself a drink and becomes angry. He tells himself he should have hit back at the man, that the bus queue should have jumped on the man and attacked him, that if he ever sees the man again he will inflict terrible revenge. He is very angry. His wife comes home and asks what sort of a day did he have, and the man bursts into tears.

Contained within this example are all the classic features of post-traumatic stress. The attack need not have been directed at the man himself. He could have witnessed something equally distressing, such as an accident. The impact upon the man would differ according to his ability to deal with the experience and the support he received both during and after it. Equally, what happens in the future will depend upon the man's past experiences and what takes place following the incident. So, if while walking home the next day someone from the bus queue walks up to him and apologizes for not coming to his assistance and asks how he is feeling, he is likely to feel more reassured about his ability to deal with the feelings he has about the assault. If, however, while walking home he is confronted again by his assailant, who assaults him once more, and if, as is probable, no-one comes to his assistance and the man is unable to defend himself against the attack, future events will begin to reflect the uncertainty generated by the experience.

The first possibility is that the man may arm himself with a weapon to defend himself. He may try walking home using a different route. He may use a different method of transport, i.e. the bus. He may even seek another job so that he does not have to go near the scene of the attack again. In the extreme, he may refuse to leave his own home unaccompanied.

Horowitz (1986) describes the post-traumatic stress response as being a situation where the victim involuntarily re-lives the event time and time again in their own mind, often inventing different responses and endings to the attack, but always feeling the anger and fear associated with it. There is a period where they become over-vigilant and anxious about their personal safety, while trying to push the whole event out of consciousness. Whittington and Wykes (1994a) also propose that such an event is a traumatic one leaving the individual feeling highly anxious for a period of time, which in turn reduces reasoning, social functioning and self-efficacy. Further work by Whittington and Wykes (1992, 1994b) suggests that individuals who are assaulted tend to avoid further potentially assaulting situations. The same authors (Wykes and Whittington 1994) also show that nurses who are assaulted respond in exactly the same way as anyone else. What the literature in this area does not say is how many personal assaults, or how many events witnessed, i.e. self-mutilating incidents, suicidal attempts, distressing interpersonal abuse, does a nurse have to experience before the effects of post-traumatic stress response start to occur.

Of course, it would be impossible to provide such an answer, for just as each event is experienced differently by each partici-pant so too are its effects. It is possible that for some nurses the effects begin immediately, while for others never at all, and it is the difference between these two groups which poses the question, 'Are there ways to prepare an individual to deal effec-tively with such stress responses?' We will return to this question during the macro section of the chapter, but first think again about the man attacked in the above example. What if this had been a nurse, assaulted by a client, and instead of the bus queue, other members of staff witnessed the event without really coming to her assistance, providing only superficial support afterwards. Is it likely that the nurse would feel aggrieved by their actions and those of the client involved? Is it possible that she might take the same actions as the man in the original example, becoming angry and resentful, but re-living the event and being anxious and fearful about it. Is it possible that, as Whittington and Wykes (1994a) suggest, she will question her efficacy, misinterpret the intentions and behaviours of others, lose the ability to interact appropriately, and find it increasingly difficult to make rational and logical decisions about the whole event? Both Riggs *et al.* (1992) and Hendin (1992) would say, yes.

Riggs *et al.* examined the feelings of female crime victims and found that there appeared to be a direct correlation between the amount of anger that the victim felt and the degree of post-traumatic stress they experienced. Hendin, by contrast, looked at the risk of suicide for military veterans who suffered post-traumatic stress, and felt that those who showed guilt over actions in combat were more likely to attempt suicide than those who did not. While nursing is not combat, the matter of self-efficacy remains a key factor for both groups of professionals. This view is supported by the work of Smith and Hart (1994) who saw self-efficacy as a major factor for nurses having to deal with high levels of personal threat, while Roberts (1991) and Ryan and Poster (1991) were concerned that such issues were considered when exploring the nature of nurses' responses to psychiatric emergencies.

Nurses who experience assault, or who witness distressing events, either regularly or in a one-off situation, are just as at risk of suffering the effects of post-traumatic stress as any other member of the public, including the clients who experience PEs from a different standpoint. The effects of violence are not altered because of a person's occupation. Such effects include the inability to make decisions or prioritize effectively, lack of concentration, reductions in self-confidence, self-efficacy and self-esteem, being over-cautious, becoming agitated, tearful and distressed, not sleeping or eating properly, failing to maintain social contacts, being fearful, frightened, lonely and clinically depressed. This is supported by considerable scientific evidence (Dionne-Proulz and Pepin 1993, Ryan and Poster 1993, Corless 1994, Jamieson 1994).

It is crucial to nurses' support mechanisms that they recognize the impact such stress may have upon their ability to carry out their work satisfactorily, but so too is the fact that it may be possible to counteract the effects of PTS. The feelings of anger experienced by the man attacked in the example, and the subsequent tearful response when the barriers come down and the whole event is re-lived in all its fearful entirety, the inability to come to terms with what happened, the challenge to self-confidence and capabilities, the fear of further attack, are all features of PTS that a nurse may experience following a PE. The failure experienced by the man (or the nurse), as discussed in the next two sections of the chapter, may not relate so much to what they did but to what others did to support them.

The micro issue: effects on the individual

Some of the effects of stress have already been mentioned, but the full list is considerably larger. In reality there is no limit to what can happen but usually the adverse effects inhibit the person's ability to function as an independent, self-satisfying individual. Life is restricted, as are alternatives, and memories of events are painful and distressing. Perhaps as significant are the knock-on effects these have upon the person's ability to interact with others. Either the only thing that can be discussed is the event or situation causing the distress, or the event is not discussed at all. In the first case those who come into contact with the person may find it difficult to relate to what is being said, becoming embarrassed and eventually avoiding the person. In the second case the issues are never really addressed and consequently others may become confused and annoyed by the behaviour of the individual. Such a response may be exacerbated if the person is failing to do their job effectively, not taking appropriate responsibilities, consistently making small mistakes and refusing to accept help or support. Within a nursing setting such responses may extend to the relationships with clients, and it is not difficult to imagine the difficulties this may generate, not least of all in the development of future potential PEs.

Farmer *et al.* (1992) interviewed 43 male underground train drivers whose trains had killed or injured individuals – usually as the result of suicide attempts. In their case a major consideration was the increase in the amount of sick leave the men had taken since the events. In another study, Freyne and O'Connor (1992) looked at the psychological effects upon six male adult prisoners of witnessing, or being friends with, prisoners who had attempted to hang themselves, in one case successfully. Half of the group developed symptoms of PTSD, while a seventh attempted suicide by hanging.

In a paper more closely related to nursing Mericle (1993) describes a similar situation occurring when a nursing colleague commits suicide. Miller and Basoglu (1991) and Riggs *et al.* (1992) describe similar effects, with the Riggs study paying particular attention to the amount of anger expressed by victims of attacks or violence. The Hendin (1992) paper, as discussed earlier, deals specifically with another major factor, that of guilt. These studies highlight the possible impact that a PE may have upon the individual, though in the same way that each event will affect people in different ways, so too it must be remembered that not all responses to a PE need be as dramatic as full PTSD.

The most likely responses are those which affect the individual's ability to function effectively. These include the following:

- Fear of being attacked again.
- Feeling rejected by the client.
- Anger at the client.
- Worry about what colleagues will think about you.
- Being frightened of losing control.
- Losing confidence in your ability to carry out similar work.
- Not being able to think about anything else (uncontrollably re-living the event).
- Not feeling ready to carry out work expected of you.
- Feeling that you have let people down.
- Feeling guilty.
- Losing your sense of humour.
- Feeling that you have failed.

If these feelings and beliefs are not dealt with satisfactorily relatively quickly after the event they will begin to have secondary effects upon both personal and professional competence. Such features may include the following:

- Reduction in confidence.
- Reduction in the amount of work undertaken.
- Reduction in social contact.
- Reduction in ability to involve yourself in therapeutic discussion.
- Reduction in the use of new ideas.
- Increase in personal control measures, resulting in a reduction in the client's involvement in care decisions.
- Increase in repetitious actions, thus providing you with artificial security.
- Increase in fear of further attack.
- Increase in doubts about your own abilities.
- Increase in suspicion that others are waiting for you to make mistakes.

There is no evidence to show that the severity of a violent or disturbing incident will influence the nature of the response to it. Thus, just because one nurse has to witness a particularly distressing self-mutilating incident it does not mean that his/her response to it cannot be as dramatic as that of a nurse badly beaten by a client. Similarly, the nurse who is beaten may recover much quicker from his/her experience than the nurse witnessing the self-mutilation. So, not only does the severity of the incident not influence the severity of the response, it also does not have any real bearing on the recovery process. This is dependent upon something else.

The recovery process

Just as the professional application of therapeutic skills to a PE involves several stages, as with the AIRS framework, so too the recovery process from such events may follow a certain regular pattern. Resolution of the feelings generated by such experiences can only occur once the individual has come to terms with the way they have affected them. Making sense of those feelings is a crucial issue, but coming to terms with their significance for them as an individual is even more important. This book cannot help individuals with the remedial work needed to make sense of their own feelings, putting them into context and then relating them to the personal experiences of a traumatic PE. What it can do, however, is state the obvious, which is, that the process of recovery cannot usually be undertaken in isolation. People need people. Nurses are no different. The recovery process is facilitated by others being prepared to provide appropriate support for their colleagues, instead of walking away and ignoring them (Morle 1990, Harvey 1992, Holland and Leiba 1993).

All those involved in a PE should undergo a debriefing session. This can take any format. It can be carried out by those involved in the PE itself, though it is always advisable to have someone present who was not involved, who can therefore be more objective about the event. It can be undertaken by a clinical supervisor. This ought to be someone acting in a clinical, as opposed to a managerial, role. It may be difficult for a nurse to admit to someone who controls their employment contract that that they have difficulty working with a certain client or group of clients. The purpose of clinical supervision is to support those working in clinical contact, to identify weaknesses and develop them into strengths. It is also about supporting people when they feel they may have failed.

The debriefing may not be as formal as this. Nurses involved in a PE ought actively to seek colleagues with whom they can share their experiences. This will usually mean identifying someone on the clinical team, and it does not have to be another nurse, whom they trust sufficiently to be honest and supportive, but who will be able to be constructive about their support. In other words, it is not about waiting till you go to the pub in the evening to tell others what you have been involved in during the day, to get their support for the way you feel as a method of reinforcing your own actions, or the anger you feel towards your clients or colleagues. For it is not about simply telling someone what happened, though that is a good place to begin. It is about making sense of what happened, and this requires an understanding on the part of the person acting as the debriefer of the circumstances in which the PE took place and the various events which impacted upon it. It also requires skill in active listening, and the desire to really help the nurse come to terms with their feelings about the event, rather than simply rationalizing them all away.

Why does a session have to be so formal? Many clinical staff use their wives, husbands or life partners as the debriefer. Usually this ritual takes place in the home kitchen and takes the line of one person re-living the day's events to the other while the evening meal is being prepared. While this is a good place to begin, especially if the other also has knowledge of the work the care professional does, such an approach is only superficial because it fails to resolve the difficulties associated with being critical and constructive following such events. A spouse or partner may be more likely to be sympathetically supportive, thus again reinforcing the belief that everything the person feels or believes is correct. And conversely the lack of support by a spouse or partner in a relationship that is going through problems may make it even more difficult for the nurse to cope with his or her feelings. In extreme cases nurses' reactions to a PE may be be loaded by 'bad' feelings about a crisis in their personal lives. Once these beliefs become deep-seated it becomes even more difficult to deal effectively with them, and the effects upon personal and professional activities identified above become even more difficult to tackle.

Whitfield (1994) talks of restoring psychological equilibrium as the process by which an individual nurse recovers from serious events such as a PE. This is a useful term because it describes the notion that the nurse is attempting to reach a stable relationship both with themselves and what is going on around them. Sometimes it takes the actions of others to bring this about.

The support process

What if the nurse does not seek support? If nurses do not seek the support of others following these events it is important their colleagues are prepared to take responsibility for doing so. Senior nurses ought to be aware of the pressures on their staff and should make time in their own schedules to debrief following a PE. Similarly it may be the senior nurse who is involved in the event and someone also needs to be aware of their needs. No nurse should take part in a PE and then not receive proper support afterwards.

Where should the session take place? The debriefing itself ought to take place away from the main clinical area, and the staff involved in it should not be interrupted. Where possible, other staff may need to cover while the process is undertaken. Such things as telephones, pagers etc. should not be responded to. The time taken will vary depending on the support needed. However, it is important that support does not follow along the lines of 'Are you OK?' – end of support! Of course, if the incident has taken place within a community setting and the nurse has had to drive somewhere to get to the debriefing session it may be easier to chose a convenient site. However, in such circumstances where the PE was particularly violent and/or the nurse has called for help it may be necessary to undertake the session in the car, because the nurse is in no fit state to drive until it has taken place.

What goes on in the session? Usually a recap of the event itself, beginning with the events which led up to it, what happened during it, how it was resolved and the support processes used to help the client afterwards. Others may have been involved, and not just healthcare professionals, so their part in the proceeding will need to be discussed and assessed. The AIRS framework can be used to structure the session; thus the assessment looks at what happened before the event, the client's behaviour, the nurse's behaviour, the actual event and the nature of the PE. The intervention will explore what was done to bring the PE to a conclusion and reduce the amount of emotional tension being experienced by the client. The resolution will concentrate on how the nurse managed to bring the PE to an end and provide the client with an acceptable opt-out of the event, and finally the support will cover what is happening now to ensure that the client is recovering from the event and has the same opportunities to make sense of the PE as the nurse is receiving.

What happens after the session? This will depend on the impact of the PE on the nurse. While it does not always follow that exposure to more and more of these events enables the nurse to deal more effectively with them, nor does it follow that the degree of recovery from the event can be easily assessed. A ten minute debriefing ought to be a minimum for anyone involved in a serious PE, irrespective of whether they say they need to or not. Longer sessions may occur as a result of what is said, or perhaps not said, during them. Support after the session will be something determined by the nature of the nurse's response. If the nurse appears to be coping well, then perhaps this will be an end to it. If recovery is not so obvious then further discussion time may be needed, or perhaps a rescheduling of the nurse's work. In extreme cases the nurse may need to be sent home from work and ultimately take some time off. The debriefing session is the method used to make the assessment of the nurse's needs.

What should the session achieve? Six things.

Firstly, the opportunity for the nurse to discuss the event in a controlled and rational way, gaining critical and constructive support for his/her involvement in it.

Secondly, to explore the professional issues that the event raises and to find alternatives that may be used in future practice.

Thirdly, to assess the impact of the event upon the nurse's ability to perform his/her clinical actions.

Fourthly, to demonstrate that colleagues are concerned about the nurse's welfare.

Fifthly, to provide a forum in which feelings of failure, rejection, anger and guilt can be addressed safely.

Finally, to act as the medium through which long-term support, guidance and possibly counselling can be both identified and actioned. It could be argued that the session had one more immediate purpose, that of giving the nurse the time out to regain composure and prepare him/herself for a return to client contact.

The macro issue: effects on the organization

If individuals within a work environment do not feel safe or competent to carry out their work, or sufficiently supported to be able to work effectively, it stands to reason that the performance of that workforce will be affected. A short-term reduction in care quality can be redressed quite quickly, but the longer this continues the more individuals see this practice as the norm, and therefore acceptable. Consistent with this is not just a reduction in the care quality, but other stress-related factors such as staff sickness and burnout. Practice developments will not take place, industrial relations deteriorate and generally the morale of the care teams and the clients is poor.

Taking this one step further, people will not wish to work in such an area; thus staff leave and it becomes harder to recruit replacements. So, we have an unhappy, stressed, and over-worked care team, working with a similarly unhappy, stressed and ultimately neglected client group. Just the right sort of environment for a violent or aggressive PE to take place, and one in which it is unlikely to be dealt with effectively, either from a client's perspective or a nursing one (Jamieson 1994).

Dionne-Proulz and Pepin (1993) argue that organizational, rather than individual, role factors are far more influential in the development of stress-related responses to crisis. Tommasini (1992) also found that the setting up of a staff support group to deal with the impact of PEs in a specialist psychiatric unit had just as much effect upon the work environment as it did upon the nursing and care group. This finding was supported by both Cassells *et al.* (1990) and Corless (1994).

It makes sense to support the care team, that is obvious, but how can this be achieved?

The following are a series of ideas and approaches which, singularly, may not have a great impact upon the PE itself, but collectively may provide an environment in which it can be dealt with professionally and effectively.

Staff support mechanisms

Johnson (1982) identified four key areas of an on-going staff support mechanism: practical help, sharing experiences, shared information and the stimulation of ideas. All these can be achieved within the one-to-one sessions described for individual staff support following a PE. Providing time for those involved in such activities has to be of prime importance for managers. Even if it is not possible to build any other support structure into the care process this one acknowledgement of the need to make both time and space for people undergoing stress-ful pressure within the workplace can make a great difference to the care team's perception of corporate support. Management are sometimes accused of not understanding the complexities of client contact, but they can appreciate what being hit means.

Agreeing to support these sessions, both in manpower terms and financially, is a recognition of the importance of the work being undertaken.

Clinical supervision

Individuals need to be able to trust the people with whom they share their clinical difficulties, be they success or failures. The support mechanisms needed to help someone directly after a PE may begin with a cup of coffee and a quiet, supportive word from a friend, but it needs to progress to something more formal and structured. The continuity offered by a realistic clinical supervision model, one based upon clinical rather than managerial criteria, is an excellent forum for this work to take place. In developing clinical supervision programmes, managers need to recognize that the contract between the nurse and the supervisor may also include special time out as necessitated by a PE. They must also recognize that the nurse–supervisor confidentiality and relationship may be the main keys to the successful resumption of any post-event stress reaction experienced by the nurse.

Educational developments

The obvious choice here is for on-going experiential workshops to help deal with interpersonal conflict. These would be devised around the needs of the care group, rather than following the traditional pattern of educationalists and managers deciding between them what it was that the care team needed.

It is important that other aspects of the PE are catered for. This includes control and restraint courses, dealing with aggressive incidents and in particular realistic and effective practical help for people who find themselves being threatened or abused. Certainly there is evidence to show that once staff feel that they are able to defend themselves properly in difficult situations, they tend to take less risks, and place themselves in less dangerous situations than if they felt more threatened. The self-efficacy issue has been raised several times in this book (Chapters 2, 5 and 6 particularly), and certainly nurses' confidence is derived from a whole series of factors, not least knowing what to do and how to do it. Taking risks does not appear to be part of self-efficacy (Goodykoontz and Herrick 1990, Holmstrom 1990, Collins 1994).

Professional support groups

Professional support groups meet at regular intervals to discuss matters affecting the work patterns of its members. Most of these groups are relatively small, unidisciplinary and attendance is voluntary. They do not meet to discuss specific topics, but are there to support their members should they have particular problems. While they can be a good forum to discuss matters arising from a PE, they are not necessarily the best place to seek an objective overview of what happened and what lessons can be learnt.

In certain clinical environments it is possible to convene critical incident groups who will meet following a major event, such as a plane or train crash where the victims were cared for by the department (Burns and Holland 1991). Whitfield (1994) describes the characteristics of such a multidisciplinary group within an A&E setting, but equally, following a major PE, similar groups could be convened to ensure that all staff had the opportunity to 'off-load' their part of the event. The main purpose of these groups is not to make people talk about what happened but to explore both the sequence of events and the effects it had upon those involved.

If professional support groups are to be incorporated into the structure it is important that they deal with issues relating specifically to clinical contact. The group should be lead by a professional who has credibility for all those who take part, and there is some evidence to suggest that an outside facilitator may be the best person to run such groups. If PEs are to be the subject discussed it has to be realized that this forum will not provide individuals with answers to their own needs. This is a forum where general issues are discussed and where policy, procedural and strategy problems may be raised.

Research

There is much work looking at the area of aggression and violence within mental healthcare settings (Whittington and Wykes 1994b). What much of the literature recommends is that individual institutions, organizations and units explore the nature of their own incidents and make necessary provisions accordingly. The same can be said for PEs generally. Gathering data about the people involved, the times of the day, the nature of the event, the type of responses or interventions used, the support mechanisms used and the short-term effects are all helpful in making decisions about staffing levels, mix and preparation. Being aware of national initiatives is certainly one way of keeping staff up to date about alternatives, and providing the stimulus for change and professional development, but it has to be applied within a setting which is both receptive to change and appropriate for it. Providing baseline PE data would certainly be the first step in that process.

Caseload monitoring

Within a community setting there are always going to be problems associated with the size and nature of an individual practitioner's caseload. Mental health nurses working in the community, case managers working with the long-term mentally ill and carer support groups will always find that demand invariably outstrips supply. However, it is not so much the size of caseloads which is a problem here, though in truth it can cause PE problems, it is more the dependency of the caseload. The mix of clients within the caseload will determine several factors, such as contact time and therapeutic responsibilities. Where there are clients on the caseload who potentially may experience a PE, in theory these may take up more time than others. However, this is often not the case as care workers try to spread themselves evenly across their client group. Careful monitoring of clients who are at risk must be made by clinical supervisors to ensure that such clients are getting the support they need, but more importantly that the care worker is not being asked to cope with clients for whom s/he has not been prepared.

Conclusion

This chapter has considered the process of support by looking at what may happen to staff once a PE has occurred. The relationship between staff responses to stressful events and the incidence, presentation and impact of post-traumatic stress responses generally is one which cannot be ignored. While it may be true that many staff can deal with the irritating problems associated with verbal abuse, and distressing scenes of self-mutilation, it becomes harder to shift the memories of a personal physical attack, and to allow them not to influence the way you carry out your work in the future. This chapter suggests that all PEs should be treated in the same way and staff support should be offered to people whether they ask for it or not.

The micro and macro issues of PEs have been discussed in some detail. The micro, or individual, support centres around the notion that the best way to deal with a PE is to work out what really happened and to assess whether your own involvement in it was successful or not, and if not how it could have been improved. The macro, or organizational, impact of support is to ensure that the healthcare workforce is properly prepared and supported while trying to work effectively in the situations in which carers find themselves, and to provide suitable opportunities to develop those support structures based on reasoned argument and empirical evidence.

Nursing is a difficult job at the best of times. Nurses are expected to be able to deal with every aspect of human pain and suffering, and in doing so they run the risk of becoming casualties themselves. It is the responsibility of every nurse to support his/her colleagues in any way possible, both during and after situations for which they may not have been prepared, or during which they are put at risk. It is the organization's responsibility to make sure that the mechanisms for that support are in place and functioning properly. If healthcare professionals become casualties of their own work through a lack of support, either by colleagues or their employers, this is a sad indictment of the so-called caring services. More importantly, should such a situation occur, it will be the system which is the failure, not the nurse.

References

Burns, T. P. and Holland, S. C. (1991). Psychiatric response to the Clapham railcrash. *Journal of the Royal Society of Medicine*, 84(1):15–19.

Cassells, J. M., Silva, M. C. and Chop, R. M. (1990). Administrative strategies to support staff nurses as moral agents in clinical practice. *Nursing Connections*, 3(4):31–7.

Collins, J. (1994). Nurses' attitudes towards aggressive behaviour, following attendance at 'The Prevention and Management of Aggressive Behaviour Programme'. *Journal of Advanced Nursing*, 20:117–31.

Corless, R. (1994). Staff support. *Nursing Standard*, 8(23):21.

Dionne-Proulz, J. and Pepin, R. (1993). Stress management in the nursing profession. *Journal of Nursing Management*, 1(2):75–81.

Farmer, R. D., Tranah, T., O'Donnell, I. and Catalan, J. (1992). Railway suicide: the psychological effects upon drivers. *Psychological Medicine*, 22(2):407–14.

Freyne, A. and O'Connor, A. (1992). Post traumatic stress disorder symptoms in prisoners following a cell mate's hanging. *Irish Journal of Psychological Medicine*, 9(1):42– 4.

Goodykoontz, L. and Herrick, C. A. (1990). Evaluation of an inservice education programme regarding aggressive behaviour on a psychiatric unit. *Journal of Continuing Education in Nursing*, 21(3):129–33.

Harvey, P. (1992). Staff support groups: are they necessary? *British Journal of Nursing*, 1(5):256–8.

Hendin, H. (1992). 'PTSD and risk of suicide': reply. *American Journal of Psychiatry*, 149(1):143.

Holland, S. and Leiba, T. (1993). Approaching with care: violence at work. *Nursing Standard*, 7(52):3–8, 11–13.

Holmstrom, C. (1990). Nurse assault. *Canadian Journal of Psychiatric Nursing*, 31(4):6–8.

Horowitz, M. J. (1986). *Stress Response Syndromes*, 2nd edn. Aronson, NY.

Jamieson, S. (1994). Developing staff support. *Nursing Standard*, 8(28):44–6.

Johnson, R. (1982). The professional support group: a model for psychiatric clinical nurse specialists. *Journal of Psychosocial Nursing and Mental Health Services.*, 20(2):9–12.

Mericle, B. P. (1993). When a colleague commits suicide. *Journal of Psychosocial Nursing and Mental Health Services*, 31(9):11–13.

Miller, T. W. and Basoglu, M. (1991). Post traumatic stress disorder: the impact of life events on adjustment. *Integrative Psychiatry*, 7(3–4):207–15.

Morle, K. (1990). The need for staff support. *Nursing (UK): The Journal of Clinical Practice Education and Management*, 4(2):36.

Riggs, D. S., Dancu, C. V., Gershuny, B. S. and Greenberg, D. *et al.* (eds) (1992). Anger and post traumatic stress disorder in female crime victims. *Journal of Traumatic Stress*, 5(4):613–25.

Roberts, S. (1991). Nurse abuse: a taboo topic. *The Canadian Nurse*, 87(3):23–5.

Ryan, J. A. and Poster, E. C. (1991). When a patient hits you: a post assault that puts nurses first. *The Canadian Nurse*, 87(8):23–5.

Ryan, J. A. and Poster, E. C. (1993). Workplace violence: the findings of a major *Nursing Times* survey that examined nurses' experiences of assault by patients or clients. *Nursing Times*, 89(48):38–41.

Smith, M. A. and Hart, G. (1994). Nurses' responses to patient anger: from disconnecting to connecting. *Journal of Advanced Nursing*, 20:643–51.

Tommasini, N. R. (1992). The impact of a staff support group on the work environment of a speciality unit. *Archives of Psychiatric Nursing*, 6(1):40–7.

Whitfield, A. (1994). Critical incident debriefing in A&E. *Emergency Nurse*, 2(2):6–9.

Whittington, R. and Wykes, T. (1992). Staff strain and social support in a psychiatric hospital following an assault by a patient. *Journal of Advanced Nursing*, 17:480–86.

Whittington, R. and Wykes, T. (1994a). An observational study of associations between nurse behaviour and violence in psychiatric hospitals. *Journal of Psychiatric and Mental Health Nursing*, 1(2):85–92.

Whittington, R. and Wykes, T. (1994b). Violence to staff in psychiatric hospitals: are certain staff prone to be assaulted? *Journal of Advanced Nursing*, 19:219–25.

Wykes, T. and Whittington, R. (1994). Reactions to assault. In T. Wykes (ed.), *Violence and Health Care Professionals*, Chapman & Hall, London.

Suggested reading

Courage, M. M., Godgerg, K. L., Ingram, D. A., Schramm, L. L. and Hale, W. (1993). Suicide in the elderly: staying in control. *Journal of Psychosocial Nursing and Mental Health Services*, 31(7):26–31.

(What happens to nurses and carers when someone for whom they are responsible commits suicide? This paper looks at both personal and organizational effects.)

Guillory, B. A. and Riggin, O. Z. (1991). Developing a nursing support group model. *Clinical Nurse Specialist*, 5(3):170–3. (Several issues are covered within this paper which deal with the setting up of a group, including group stressors, clinical knowledge base and group outcomes.)

Joseph, S. A., Williams, R. and Yule, W. (1992). Crisis support, attributional style, coping style and post traumatic symptoms. *Personality and Individual Differences*, 13(11):1249–51. (This study asks questions about the type of support most effective for different types of coping mechanisms.)

Index